CW01511819

LIGHT UP

MIRIAM HUSSEY is a pharmacist with over a decade's experience. With extensive qualifications in integrative health and wellness, nutritional wellbeing, spirituality, yoga, meditation and mindfulness, she has a profound understanding of the real drivers of true wellbeing. Accredited with the All-Star Business Award for 'Thought Leader in Human Health and Performance', she is at the forefront of the Soul Space movement with her husband, the No. 1 bestselling author Gerry Hussey.

LIGHT UP

ENERGISE YOUR BODY

AWAKEN YOUR MIND

SUPERCHARGE YOUR SOUL

MIRIAM HUSSEY

GILL BOOKS

Gill Books
Hume Avenue
Park West
Dublin 12
www.gillbooks.ie

Gill Books is an imprint of M.H. Gill and Co.

978 07171 9719 4

Designed by Sarah McCoy
Edited by Jane Rogers
Proofread by Emma Dunne
Printed and Bound in the UK using 100% Renewable
Electricity at CPI Group (UK) Ltd
This book is typeset in Utopia Regular.

This book is not intended as a substitute for the medical
advice of a physician. The reader should consult a doctor
or mental health professional if they feel it necessary.

*The paper used in this book comes from the wood pulp of
sustainably managed forests.*

To the best of our knowledge, this book complies in full with
the requirements of the General Product Safety Regulation
(GPSR). For further information and help with any safety
queries, please contact us at productsafety@gill.ie.

A CIP catalogue record for this book is available from the
British Library.

5 4 3 2 1

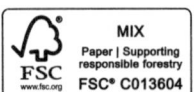

FSC
www.fsc.org

MIX
Paper | Supporting
responsible forestry
FSC® C013604

I dedicate this book to my loving husband, children and family, who have always supported and encouraged me to follow my dreams. Thank you for believing in me and for standing by my side through every challenge and triumph. This book is a testament to your unwavering love and for that, I am forever grateful.

CONTENTS

AUTHOR'S NOTE

My desire is to live a life of grace.

One that is founded on gratitude and huge respect for the blessings that are in my life and the tiny miracles that exist in every moment.

To live a life of grace is to accept, not judge, to take responsibility, not blame, to live a life of defencelessness, not preach or demand. It's to trust life and the journey and to learn to live comfortably in the uncertainty, leaning into the knowingness that our greatest opportunities often lie in this uncertain and energetic space. It's to not strive or resist, just surrender and live with ease.

It's to learn to serve humanity and offer my love and assistance for the greater good of this world. It's to live a life steeped in God and his teachings and to understand the unity and oneness of us all.

It's to not deny myself yet not glorify myself. It's to learn to live authentically with humility and honesty and to come home to my soul within, so that I can live a life of ease and grace and by doing so become a beacon of light for this world.

My mission is to keep finding the light, no matter how dark things get; it is to spread light in whatever capacity I can; and it is to empower people to connect to the divine light and reignite their own inner sparkle. My mission is to help people's hearts glow again, to let their souls illuminate with an unshakeable shine and help our world expand in the emanating ripples of these glimmers, enabling us all to collectively LIGHT UP.

INTRODUCTION

It's 4:30 am. I step outside into the cold, and immediately want to retreat back to the warmth of indoors, back to security. So many times in my past, I would have done exactly that, but not this time. This time something is different, something inside me feels different, something is moving, rising. After years of running away, suppressing and denying, this is different – I'm tired of running, fed up of suppressing and, in this moment, there's a new glimmer of courage that is not allowing me to go back.

I make my way to the bench on the cliff, the bench that will become my bench of hope, my bench of dreams, my bench of truth. I sit and listen to the wind, to the magnificent roar of the sea as the waves crash against the rocks far below. It's perfectly dark, yet I can see more clearly than ever.

These last few days I have been on retreat in Dzogchen Beara, a Tibetan Buddhist retreat centre on the Beara Peninsula in County Cork, in south-west Ireland. I have allowed myself to be totally open, truly honest and, at times, painfully raw. This retreat is different; it isn't a retreat to simply top up on self-care, it is a retreat to unravel the essence of who I am and to come home to my heart.

As I sit there taking in the cacophony of sounds, the universe is providing the backdrop, and whatever is rising within me is coming from my deepest truth. After years of it being drowned out, I am not letting anything distract me from its calling.

From the outside things looked 'good': I was a qualified pharmacist, educated at the prestigious Royal College of Surgeons; I had a highly paid career, relationships that were loving and safe – all the ingredients that the world says make a great life. Yet, here on this bench in the darkness of the early morning, I had more clarity than ever: this might make someone else happy and content, but there was a voice deep within telling me that this wasn't nourishing my soul, this wasn't setting me free.

Leaving the safe and familiar is made a little easier if we have a plan B: a clear plan and a guarantee it can work. I didn't have any of those. Plan A was the safe, the familiar, the known. Plan B was a blank canvas, with zero safety, zero guarantees, zero roadmaps. But, as I listened to that voice rising within me, I kept hearing that my plan B also had zero limits. **Sometimes in life we don't have to know where we are going or what the end looks like, we just need to know that where we are isn't right.**

Michelangelo believed the sculpture of *David* was already present within the block of marble; his role was merely to chip away the excess material around it, chip away everything that wasn't David, which would then reveal the statue within. Similarly, in life, we might not know what our 'statue' is or where our path will lead, but we know that staying where we currently are isn't working. It is not healthy, it is not nourishing and it is not authentic. Oftentimes, coming home to wholeness is not about actively pursuing our true self; sometimes it's as simple as slowly shedding everything that is not truly us. Sitting on that bench, I was absolutely clear that every fibre of my being was telling me to leave plan A – the prescribed life, the ordinary – and step bravely into uncertainty. For the first time in my life, I was ready to answer the call.

I knew what I had to do, I knew how hard it would be, the resistance I would meet, that it wouldn't make sense to people, but I also knew that not doing it would mean never being willing to find my truth, to honour my heart and follow my soul's script.

I stood up from the bench and I was shaking. I knew my life was about to change for ever. As the wind and the waves continued to roar, I could hear the little Miriam within me beginning to roar too. For years she had denied her true essence, suppressed her real identity and believed that her dreams were silly. She believed her light was not worthy to be seen. As I stared at the horizon, I saw a glimmer of first light, a faint drop of orange and pink unveiling itself against the black sky – the gracious gap between the night's rawness and the dawn's brightness, the space between the 'no longer' and the 'not yet'. As the sun rose, I too felt a surge of heat, an inner glow rising within me. I felt as if each breath I took was stoking the embers of the fire, fanning the flames to ignite the inner confidence and courage I knew I would need in the weeks and months ahead as I embarked on this journey, a journey that would involve great change. I felt scared, but I also felt a deep knowingness. A surrendering wave washed over my body. My shoulders dropped, my chest unclasped its grip of fear, and as I wiped away the last of my tears, I was embraced by what felt like a warm hug. Call it the universe, God, divine energy, but in that moment, I felt a God-like energy was cloaking me, both in an armour to face what I needed to and a protective blanket to wrap me up and keep me safe. I knew that I was going to be okay and that all would be well. I was taking little Miriam by the hand and telling her, **'I see you, I hear you, I've got you, I love you.'** I was giving her back her voice, I was honouring her truth and I was ready to let the world see her incredible light. The pretending was over, the denial had ceased, and while I had no idea what path lay ahead, I knew it would be a path of greater freedom, passion and truth, where I would dare to dream without limits, dare to be without distraction and dare to live without regrets.

These transitional shifts in life are like growing pains: they are uncomfortable and unpleasant, but with time they yield our greatest growth, transformation and liberation. In this book, I will share my journey with you, I will open my heart and be as honest and authentic as I can. I will share what I believe to be wholesome information. I dare not preach, but simply hold space for you to do your own inner reflective work, so that you, too, can come home to your deepest truths and light up to live a life of greater joy, vitality, ease and grace.

The integrative journey

Growing up in the west of Ireland, I was always drawn to the health and wellness space. Anything to do with the human body excited me, and from as early as I can remember I knew I was destined to live a life that would be focused on health and wellbeing. When I was 14 years old, my mam handed me a book that would forever change my life: Louise Hay's *You Can Heal Your Life*. It was my greatest companion during my teenage years and became even more influential in my college years and beyond. The book's messages sparked a huge interest in the power of the mind–body connection, how deeply integrated our entire system is, how everything we think about, feel and perceive has a direct impact on our health and wellbeing. It led me to explore the realm of energy, God or frequency, and the impact that something greater than ourselves has on our lives. I was enthralled by the idea that when we are plugged into this universal flow, it is like a supercharged vital-force connection that enables us to feel empowered, aligned, regulated and healthy. Ever since then, my deep passion for lifestyle medicine and integrative health has been growing, evolving and expanding.

My journey into the world of health began when I trained to become a pharmacist. I learned so much along my pharmacy journey, but my passion for a more holistic, whole-body and integrative approach to health was niggling at me. Ten years working as a community-based pharmacist witnessing 'a pill for every ill' approach opened my eyes to the way we treat sickness. It made me look more deeply into the true meaning of wellness and beyond the one-dimensional model of treating the symptom.

I received my greatest teachings working on the front line in the community, where extraordinary lessons and learnings unfolded every day. I had the space to really observe human behaviour, lifestyle patterns and the impact of what a lack of ease can do. It can be absorbed into our bodies and spill over into our souls, and vice versa; when a soul is suppressed, the negativity can ripple into our minds and bodies, creating a lack of harmony or balance, impacting the amount of ease, peace and happiness we hold in our lives.

This is where I began to see emerging patterns and how people's lifestyles and daily habits were impacting their well-being. I noticed the alarming rise in chronic diseases (such as diabetes, obesity, cardiovascular disease), cancer, autoimmune diseases, depression, anxiety, arthritis and chronic pain. According to the World Health Organization (WHO), chronic diseases are currently the major cause of death among adults in almost all countries. The toll is projected to increase by a further 17 per cent in the next 10 years.

The WHO states that chronic diseases are not passed from person to person; they are of long duration and generally slow progression. What this means is that chronic disease is not passed on like a flu or a virus; neither does it just fall out of the sky and hit you on the head. Chronic disease presents as a result of years of compounding lifestyle factors that bubble up to the surface. The body eventually says 'Enough!' **The little things we do every day are either creating a future of greater health, vitality and abundance of life-force energy, or they are creating a future of ill health and disease**. I share this not to frighten or startle you, but to empower you with the knowledge that by making small, daily lifestyle tweaks, we can impact the power of our future happiness and health.

I also began to feel that I was working not in a healthcare system but in a 'sick-care' system – a reactive model of care instead of a preventive model. People generally only came to my pharmacy when they were unwell, and often when it was too late, not as a place to get well or stay well. This greatly upset me, as I knew deep within that there is more to health than just treating the symptoms of illness. I felt that our current model of care is somewhat flawed because it addresses only the symptom, and not the root cause, like placing a Band-Aid on the disease but never actually addressing the source of what caused the problem in the first place.

I like to use the analogy of a fire. Let's say a fire starts in a building and all the fire alarms go off, and when the fire brigade arrive they just turn off the fire alarms but never actually find the source of the fire. This is similar to what I believe we are doing in our modern world of healthcare. Our body is constantly trying to communicate with us through signs and symptoms – headaches, rashes, digestive pain, discomfort, reflux, mouth ulcers, cold sores, to name just a few. In many cases, if we can become still enough, quiet enough and curious enough to truly listen, feel and become attuned to these symptoms, we could better handle them, heal and come back into alignment by altering certain life-style measures. The fast-paced, constantly plugged-in way of our modern world, where stress has become way too 'normal' and is fuelled by ultra-processed foods and beverages, is directly worsening the situation. It is not only keeping us locked in a stressed state, it is also hindering us from truly becoming present, slowing down and listening to the gentle whispers, nudges and sensations of our souls.

Every sensation in the body is information – inform-ation from our deepest self, our higher self or our soul. Information from our heart, which holds our deepest desires, dreams and emotions; information from our minds, our thoughts, our inner narratives and stories; and inform-ation from our physiology – from our cells, our organs, our hormones, our gut. If we don't listen when these signs are gentle whispers, they can elevate into giant roars or full-blown wipeouts that often present in the form of burnout, a serious diagnosis or some form of chronic disease. The word 'disease' can be broken down into 'dis-ease', or a lack of ease and harmony within oneself, whether on a physical, mental or spiritual level.

Of course there is a place for medicine: it can be life-saving and we are truly blessed to have it in our world. But I believe an integrated approach is key. One that is balanced and one that is open to working with all modalities for the good of the whole person. As we move through this book, I will be taking you on an integrative journey, which involves the unity of body, mind and soul. I will share my lessons, learnings and beliefs, as best I can, which I hope will help you on your journey towards greater health, peace and joy.

We will explore the integrative approach of the mind, body and soul and the ripple effect concept, where we view life as three circles, the outer layer or circle representing the physical body, the middle layer or circle representing the mind and the inner circle symbolising the soul – which is our inner essence, our spark of light, who we truly are. When the soul is not 'lit up', distress signals are sent out into the mind impacting our thoughts, our emotions and our feelings. This then sends ripples into the body, causing dysregulation within our nervous system, resulting in imbalance and the manifestation of symptoms, ailments or dis-ease.

But first, it is important that we identify the root causes of our discomfort and work towards bringing balance and harmony back into our lives. This can be achieved through using simple yet powerful lifestyle tools and integrative health techniques that address you as a whole person. Your mind, emotions, thoughts. Your breath, nervous system, energy field. Your past, present and future. Your thought patterns and beliefs. Your stress, your sleep, your ability to relax, repair and rest. Your why. Your soul's purpose, passion and meaning. Your heart's desires, dreams and visions. Your relationships with yourself and others, your traumas, your fears, your aspirations and hopes, your gratefulness and appreciation, your sense of faith and optimism, your nutritional wellbeing, hydration, your hidden habits and tendencies, your career, your choices, your daily habits and behaviours, your movement and exercise, your everything. Because everything you are and everything you do creates everything you become.

When you open your heart to let love flow in (as well as out) and dissolve the barriers of fear and self-doubt, and when you listen to your inner soul's calling, it will take you on an unimaginable journey. A journey inward to the source of all that truly matters. A journey of truths that will involve embracing all of life's dualities, the perceived glory as well the uncertainty and messiness. The dark, the light, the pain, the power, the burdens, the bliss. All these life experiences deepen and enrich our human evolution so that we can explore the incredible strength, wisdom and light that lies within. **This journey can be tumultuous at times, but I believe it is always worth it. This journey inward to awaken to your inner pharmacy carries potency to ignite vitality, life-force energy, fulfilment and joy.**

This voyage will untangle you, both physically and emotionally, and will set your soul free to live a life that is more aligned to your truths, your core values and your deepest desires. When embarking on this adventure we call life, we must be prepared to let go of things that no longer serve us, to step into our light and illuminate the divine-like qualities that reside in us. We must dig deep and draw on our internal well of courage to grant ourselves the permission to show up for ourselves, to honour our needs, to value our innate sense of self, and we must be willing to befriend ourselves in a whole new way.

Life is for living. Sometimes we just need to get out of our own way and let the universal tides carry us forward. As well as practical tips and tools, I hope this book will give you the support, encouragement, compassion and space to help you energise your body, awaken your mind and supercharge your soul.

It's time to LIGHT UP.

BODY, MIND, SOUL REFLECTION

Welcome to the body, mind and soul reflection. This is designed to help you gain insights into your overall wellbeing by assessing how your body, mind and soul are interconnected. Please take some time to complete the questionnaire thoughtfully and honestly so as to get the most aligned and accurate results. Your responses will help you identify areas of strength and areas for improvement, ultimately leading to a healthier and more balanced life. Take your time to answer each question and give yourself a score of one for each Yes and zero for each No.

When you've finished, tally up your score to see how you fare in achieving a balanced state of wellbeing. Please be compassionate with yourself – remember, we are all human and no one's perfect. Use this practice as an insightful opportunity for self-reflection and personal growth as you embark on this journey to harmonise your body, mind and soul. So grab a pen, find a quiet space, and let's dive in!

Body

Statement	Response (Yes/No)
1. Do you wake up feeling refreshed?	
2. Do you consistently get somewhere between 7 and 9 hours' sleep per night?	
3. Do you exercise regularly (i.e. 30 mins x 5 times a week [150 minutes] of moderate-intensity exercise or 75 minutes of vigorous exercise per week) and include movement breaks every hour if in a sedentary desk job?	
4. Do you consistently maintain a healthy diet even when you are busy at work; can you say you eat at least 5–7 portions of fruit and vegetables every day?	
5. Do you keep yourself well hydrated (i.e. drink 1.5–2 litres of water per day)?	
6. Do you recognise the signs when you are getting stressed or burnt out and do you take action to regulate your nervous system when out of balance?	
7. Do you take regular breaks during the day to renew and recharge your energy?	
8. Do you feel you have enough energy to sustain your day-to-day activities?	
9. Do you consume less than 3 cups of tea/coffee a day?	
10. Do you have at least 4–5 alcohol-free days a week?	
11. Are you a non-smoker?	

Mind

Statement	Response (Yes/No)
1. Do you recognise the signs when you are getting anxious, overwhelmed or have racing thoughts?	
2. Do you take action to rebalance and relax yourself when you are getting overwhelmed?	
3. Do you have people you can talk to about problems and find comfort in their companionship?	
4. Do you switch off in the evenings and at weekends?	
5. Do you feel confident in your ability to achieve your best performance outcomes each day?	
6. Do you ask for help when you need it?	
7. Can you easily focus on one thing at a time and avoid getting distracted during the day?	
8. Do you engage in mental fitness practices every day (e.g. meditation, visualisation, gratitude, mirror work, deep breathing, positive affirmations, journalling)?	
9. Do you feel you direct your emotions (e.g. anger, sadness, frustration, boredom) in a healthy way?	
10. Do you regularly stop to savour your accomplishments and blessings and express appreciation of yourself and others?	
11. Do you feel focused, calm, composed and alert under pressure or during busy times?	

Soul

Statement	Response (Yes/No)
1. Do you feel passionate about what you do?	
2. Do you have a sense of meaning and purpose in your life?	
3. Do you prioritise time for fun, laughter and the activities that you truly enjoy in life?	
4. Do you spend regular time with the people you love?	
5. When you are with family and friends, do you feel truly present and engaged with them?	
6. Do you allocate your time and energy according to what you say is most important to you?	
7. Do you regularly get fresh air, spend time in nature and unplug from the busyness of the world?	
8. Do you have a regular spiritual practice (e.g. meditating, yoga, deep breathing, exercise, spending time outdoors, religious practice)?	
9. Do you let go easily, surrender with grace and trust in the universe or a higher power?	
10. Do you listen to your heart and follow your gut intuitive feelings?	
11. Are you dedicated to living a life that feels true and authentic to you?	

My total score: _____

What does your score mean?

26–33   You are fully energised and aligned, lit up and
        glowing brightly.

17–25   You are somewhat energised and aligned,
           glimmering moderately.

8–16   You're fading – your light is dimming.

0–7   You're disconnected and burnt out – your light has
           gone out.

Reflections and notes

*   What are the most important areas in your life that need
    attention? What impact are these currently having on you
    and your life?

*   What is your *why*? *Why* is your health important? *Why* is
    it important for you to make changes?

*   What would be the outcome of not changing anything in
    your life? If you continued to live the way you live, work
    the way you work, eat the way you eat, drink the way you
    drink, think the way you think, what would the impact on
    your health and happiness be in 10–15 years' time? Does
    this image inspire you or not?

*   What lights you up? What is the image of yourself that you
    aspire to? What will enable you to make this vision a reality?

As you journey through the book you will be provided with
practical and simple sustainable tools that will help you make
small changes to your everyday life. Remember, Rome wasn't
built in a day – and we must start small and make gradual
daily tweaks that are sustainable and long-lasting.

I hope this book will help and support you on your
journey as you align with your vision, energise your body and
light up your soul.

BODY

Reducing stress is possibly the best thing you can do for your life. Not just for your health but also for your happiness and for the health and happiness of those around you. Unravel your tension and awaken your vitality.

CHAPTER 1

UNDERSTANDING STRESS AND FINDING CALM

The tides of life

In our daily life we are faced with so many decisions, choices, obstacles, challenges and opportunities, all of which produce a heightened level of anxiety and stress in our body. If you are experiencing stress in your life right now, perhaps you're feeling completely overwhelmed and out of your depth, perhaps you're scared, or maybe you're just completely frazzled because of that never-ending to-do list. In situations like this, our inner voice can be screeching in our ears: 'How am I not able to cope and keep up?' 'Everybody else seems to have it all together.' 'What's wrong with me?' This tug of war inside us, between what we want to do and what we can do, makes us feel like we're not good enough.

If you are feeling like this right now, *please*, this very moment, drop your shoulders, take a deep breath and understand that you are not alone. I know this place only too well, as do so many of the people I have worked with. Our fast-paced world is cheating us in a way. It is setting us up to fail. It makes us think the lights have to be turned on all the time, and if we were to switch them off, God forbid, we'd be disapproved of, rejected, unaccepted, disloyal or disliked. We'd be a failure.

It's important that we have compassion for ourselves and begin to understand that we are all feeling broken in some way as a result of our modern way of living. But I want you to know that you are not broken. You are beautifully surviving and coping, and though you might feel broken, you are not beyond repair. We need to accept that we are human, and being human means we will face adversity and challenges, we will face bereavement and loss, we will face many things that will rattle our nervous system, throw us off balance and create disharmony and stress.

Being human also means that beyond all these challenges and imperfections, we also get to experience incredible joy, love, gratitude, adventure, freedom, flow, beauty, exhilaration and so much more. It means that we can experience the duality of all the emotions that life throws at us, without getting stuck or attached to the ones that break us. We can get knocked down, but it is also within our soul's resilience and our soul's spirit to rise back up and find the light, time and time again.

I hope by reading this book, you can begin to embrace your strengths and stresses, find beauty in your imperfections and see them as opportunities for growth, healing and true transformation.

There is beauty in the imperfect, the unfinished, the new horizon. It is the imperfections that give us depth, wisdom and power and make us truly beautiful, strong and whole.

As we navigate through this chapter on stress, which I believe is one of the most important chapters in this book, I hope you will be able to understand and deconstruct some of the stresses in your life.

There have been many moments in my life when I felt like a surfer, being tossed around by huge waves that landed me on my backside on the shoreline, covered in sand, wondering where the hell I am and which side is up. Sometimes these surges come as waves; other times they are riptides that catch you unaware or tsunamis that take over your life; but having been tossed off the surfboard many times, I have had to sit myself down, truly reassess my priorities and ask myself: *What is it all about? Who am I doing this for? Is the way I'm living my life right now enabling me or hurting me? Is it creating more ease and flow and grace or more dis-ease, struggle and strain?* I've had to make many difficult decisions in my life, saying No to certain jobs, opportunities, places and things. I had to step off the surfboard for a season or two, sit on the shoreline and simply enjoy a few sunsets.

It's also important to remember that **stress isn't always bad**. It can motivate us to take action and perform at our best. It gives us the energy to get things done and the adrenaline for peak performance. An athlete needs adrenaline to give them the focus and determination to excel. Stress can help us stay focused, alert and responsive, helping us to meet deadlines and accomplish tasks efficiently. The problem with stress arises when we enter prolonged or excessive stress, also known as chronic stress, which can lead to negative physical and mental effects and a variety of health issues, which I will discuss below.

Life can be as busy and chaotic as we choose to make it. We are programmed by our subconscious beliefs and we live life according to these inherited or sometimes self-created beliefs. The belief that you have to be busy or active in order to be seen as worthy or productive was definitely a program I replayed, and I found myself tumbling in the waves because I was incapable of saying no. This left me depleted, drained, lost and burnt out. What we must realise is that when we learn to say No to certain things, we are saying Yes to ourselves. We are saying Yes to what truly matters: to more inner ease and peace, to health and happiness, to our heart's inner desires and our soul's calling.

So, let's strip it all back.

What is stress?

Stress is an internal reaction or response to an external situation. It is a natural human response that prompts us to address challenges and threats in our lives. Everyone experiences stress to some degree. The way we respond to stress, however, makes a big difference to our overall wellbeing.

Our health is being challenged like never before. Research strongly suggests that stress plays a significant role in a wide range of health issues, affecting both physical and mental wellbeing. The Centers for Disease Control and Prevention (CDC) in the US estimates that 75–90 per cent of all doctor visits are for stress-related ailments. This is an alarming figure, and it's why learning how to navigate and manage our stress in a healthy way is deeply restorative and healing for our body, mind and soul.

Stress can take centre stage in how our nervous system operates. When we experience stress, it can spread like wildfire across the body, impacting our hormones, our organs, our cells, our thinking and mood, among many other things. This can then lead to a whole host of physical symptoms and ailments. **First comes the fire (stress), then we see the flames (symptoms).**

Your nervous system is set up to protect you, to keep you safe and alive, away from danger and threat, and to ensure your body can adapt and survive in various situations. Essentially, your nervous system is constantly evaluating whether your surroundings are safe or unsafe. Every reaction it is involved in, from what job you will take or which romantic partner you choose to the release and secretion of your hormones, is influenced by the primal instinct to keep you safe. If your nervous system perceives a threat, it will initiate a series of evolutionary biological responses to ensure your survival.

Our nervous system, however, is still quite archaic, in that its perception of threat hasn't evolved to match our highly digital world. It's almost like we're trying to use a VCR to watch YouTube. The complexities of modern life can sometimes confuse this ancient programming. Our nervous system has not upgraded its software; it is still geared towards surviving in the wild and running from bears, not being stuck in traffic or staring at a screen all day. This means that it might react to the stress of work emails, financial obligations and online interactions in the way it would react to a physical threat like a predator.

This mismatch can lead to the accumulation of stress responses that are not adequately released or processed, causing them to linger in our bodies and negatively impact our health. Additionally, the constant barrage of stressors, such as notifications, emails and news updates, overwhelms our nervous system, leading to chronic stress and its associated health issues. In essence, we are using antiquated stress response mechanisms to cope with a fast-paced, high-stress lifestyle, resulting in a detrimental impact on our wellbeing. The effects of stress on our bodies can show up:

* **Mentally**, in the form of headaches, negative destructive thought patterns, low self-esteem and worth

* **Emotionally**, in the form of increased depression, low mood, anxiety, emotional eating or constant cravings

* **Physically**, in the form of increased blood pressure, increased blood sugar levels, lowered immune system, insomnia, digestive and reproductive issues, increased heart rate and respiratory rate, tense and tight muscles

* **Chemically**, in the form of the dysregulation of our stress hormones adrenaline, noradrenaline and cortisol.

Chronic stress can also worsen pre-existing health problems and might increase our cravings for and over-dependence on or use of alcohol, tobacco and other substances.

In order to understand what happens in the body when we experience stress, it's important to explain the science so that you truly understand and acknowledge how potent stress can be. In order for us to really implement changes in our lives, become less stressed and achieve greater inner ease, grace and peace, I believe it's imperative to know *why* we would advocate for less stress in the first place. So let's delve into our nervous system, as this is where all the action happens.

What is the nervous system and how does it work?

Our nervous system is made of the brain, spinal cord and nerves. It's a complex network of nerves and cells that carry messages to and from the brain and spinal cord to various parts of the body. You can think of it as the command centre of the body. It is also our greatest pharmacy, because within our nervous system lies our ability to regulate and organise our reactions and responses and our capacity to heal. **When we understand and awaken to the wisdom of our inner pharmacy by regulating our nervous system, we can begin to live a life of greater internal ease and thus external grace.**

The nervous system is like a family tree, with various branches responsible for various functions. The central nervous system (CNS) comprises the brain and the spinal cord, and the peripheral nervous system (PNS) comprises the nerves that extend from the spinal cord to the rest of the body.

The PNS is subdivided into the somatic nervous system, which is responsible for voluntary movements (the things we have conscious control over, such as walking), and the autonomic nervous system, which is responsible for involuntary movements (the things we don't have conscious control over, such as breathing and digestion).

To go deeper again, the autonomic nervous system is broken into two main pillars: the sympathetic nervous system and the parasympathetic nervous system.

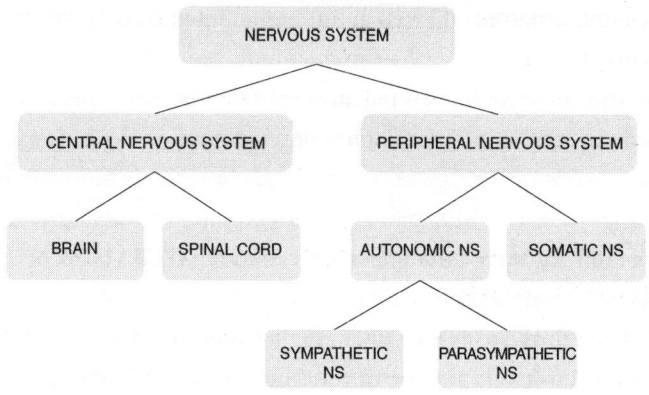

The human nervous system

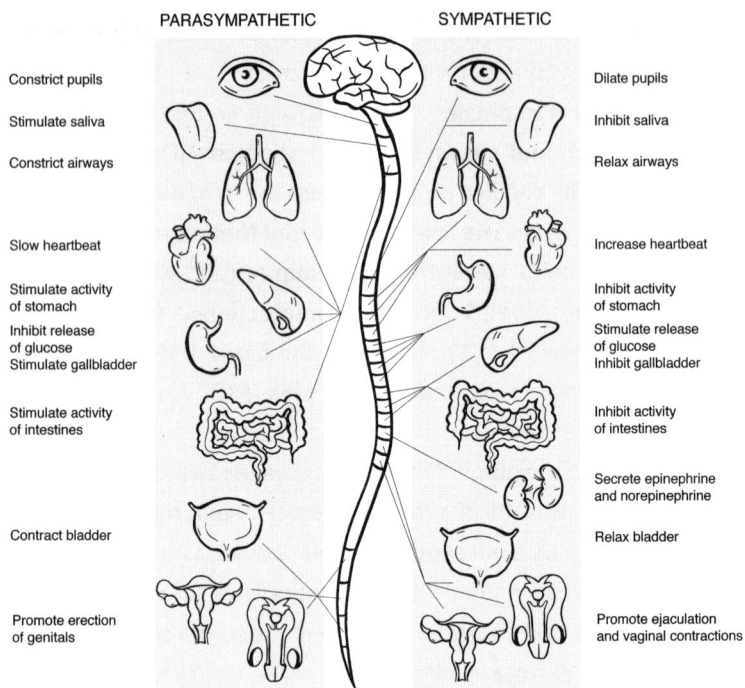

PARASYMPATHETIC   SYMPATHETIC

Constrict pupils   Dilate pupils

Stimulate saliva   Inhibit saliva

Constrict airways   Relax airways

Slow heartbeat   Increase heartbeat

Stimulate activity of stomach   Inhibit activity of stomach

Inhibit release of glucose
Stimulate gallbladder   Stimulate release of glucose
Inhibit gallbladder

Stimulate activity of intestines   Inhibit activity of intestines

    Secrete epinephrine and norepinephrine

Contract bladder   Relax bladder

Promote erection of genitals   Promote ejaculation and vaginal contractions

The parasympathetic and sympathetic nervous systems

I like to use the analogy of two siblings, John and Mary. They are very different children in temperament and character, yet both are nurtured by the same parents. Mary is busy, always on the go, always revved up and ready for action – this is the sympathetic side of the nervous system. John is more at ease, his pace is much slower, and he tends to take his time doing things – this is the parasympathetic side of the nervous system. The sympathetic nervous system, which I think of as the 'red zone', is responsible for our stress-related response (often referred to as our fight or flight response). The parasympathetic nervous system, or the 'green zone', is all about rest, digest and repair. If they are not working in harmony, or when we spend far more time on one side than the other, it leads to dysregulation and imbalance. So, in our world of busyness (including perceived busyness!), we find ourselves living in a sympathetic dominant state, which means we are in a reactive stress state *all* the time. The sympathetic nervous system is important because it's a mechanism for survival and coping with danger. If you encounter a bear, your sympathetic nervous system gets activated, flooding your body with stress hormones such as adrenaline, norepinephrine and cortisol. This enables you to either fight the bear or run the hell away. However, this survival state was only ever designed to be temporary; like a light switch, it is turned on when the threat is present, but then it is meant to be switched off when the danger disappears so that your nervous system can go back into a regulated, balanced state. We are only meant to stay in the reactive 'red zone' temporarily because our blood, our immune system and our conscious minds are all impacted dramatically when we are in a sympathetic dominant state.

Before we explore this, it is important to note that a balanced nervous system is not in a state of calm all the time. A regulated nervous system is a flexible one, and can switch between the parasympathetic and sympathetic nervous systems at times that are appropriate and necessary. It is one that can adapt easily, one that can be resilient and that can come back into harmony and coherence easily and regularly. A regulated nervous system is one where the body, mind and soul feel safe and secure. Safety is key to balancing and regulating the nervous system.

Blood flow

Through a complex system of communication from the pituitary gland in our brain to the adrenal glands in the kidneys, blood gets moved away from the centre of our body – the area from neck to buttocks where all our essential organs lie (heart, lungs, digestive organs, kidneys, spleen, liver, bladder, reproductive organs) – to our extremities (our legs and arms). This gives us the energy to either fight the bear or run away.

Our body is so intelligent that, at this moment of danger, it will say, 'Right now it's more important that I protect Miriam from this bear than it is to digest her last meal.' So my digestion is put on the back burner. Over time, or as a result of chronic and long-term stress, this can result in many digestive and gut health-related issues.

Many other functions in the body are also affected because when blood moves away from the central region, there isn't enough blood to allow the proper maintenance, repair work or cleansing action of the organs that are located there, so they get down-regulated or affected in some way. For example, your blood pressure goes up, your heart beats faster, your breathing becomes shallow and rapid, and digestion issues and gut health issues can arise. Have you ever felt like you needed to pee (kidney and bladder) or have diarrhoea (bowel) when you're nervous? I'm sure you've heard the phrase 'He wet his pants' when talking about someone who was nervous or stressed! Similarly, that wheezy feeling or butterflies in our tummy when we're anxious is a result of the blood being squeezed away from those areas. They are a physical manifestation of a stress response.

Immune system

When the body goes into stress mode, our immune system is also affected. If stress is acute (short term), it can temporarily enhance immune responses by activating immune cells. However when stress is chronic (long term) it suppresses immune function, leading to increased inflammation and greater susceptibility to illness.

For example, if there's a bacterial infection in your body, the body will *always* scan your environment to assess its safety and try to protect you from danger. However, if there's a huge threat (or perceived threat) within your nervous system, the body will decide that keeping Miriam alive is a far better option than fighting off a bacterial infection, because the bacterial infection won't be an issue if Miriam isn't alive. Our nervous system will always choose survival first, so our immune system gets put on the back burner.

A powerful example of this is seen following an organ transplant. In this situation, hormones released during periods of stress (glucocorticoids) are given to suppress the patient's immune system and prevent rejection of the new 'foreign' organ. This highlights how stress hormones shut down our immune response.

The conscious mind

Another area that's massively affected when we go into stress mode is our conscious mind. It gets shut down and so we are less able to make aligned, informed and correct decisions. When you are in a stressful state, the threat stops you thinking clearly. You become reactive and make erratic decisions that impact your life. This is because when we are in a stressful state, the blood moves from the more developed part of the brain (the prefrontal cortex, the area of the brain that's associated with logical thinking, planning, organisation, creativity and imagination) to the less developed or 'reptilian' brain (amygdala), which responds to fears, threats or conflict, and plays a role in controlling basic survival instincts that impact things like heart rate, breathing and blood pressure.

For example, during a heated argument with a loved one, stress levels increase, causing blood flow to be redirected away from the logical thinking part of the brain, which can lead to impulsive and less conscious actions, such as saying hurtful things, getting defensive or tuning out the other person's perspective.

In this stressed-out state, we don't think as clearly under pressure, we are more reactive, and we tend to go for the quick fix. This leads us to make decisions that keep us stuck in the familiar, the old, the broken. It can stop us breaking free and exploring the imaginative, creative and expansive side of our brain where we can start new projects, begin new habits and feel brave enough to explore the world. Instead, we get locked in survival and fear mode that can keep us stuck, locked and forever imprisoned.

And so life becomes an equation. When you combine:

1. blood flowing away from the vital functions and organs of the body to the extremities;

2. the immune system being down-regulated; and

3. the conscious mind shutting down ...

what you get is an incredible concoction that contributes to many of the diseases in our modern world.

All of this seems like a lot to take in, but if you find yourself in a state of sympathetic dominance, please try not to worry – though I know that's easier said than done. But trust me, **I've seen the results**. People can transform their lives in the most incredible, achievable and sustainable ways. You don't have to be stuck here for ever. There is a way out. There is light at the end of the tunnel. Stay with me.

Stress and absenteeism: exploring the void within

Earlier I spoke of stress being an internal reaction to an external stimulus, which it often is. For example, when we lose our job, or a relationship breaks down, we experience financial stress, or lose a loved one, our responses to these situations drive stress in the body.

But there's another area that causes stress which we sometimes forget or perhaps aren't even aware of. There might be an *absence* of something in our lives that results in us feeling defeated, empty, deflated and unworthy, and stress can be a by-product of that. For example, perhaps there's an absence of fun or laughter in your life; an absence of sleep, rest or down time; or a lack of love or intimacy. These 'absences' can cause a build-up of internal anxiety or stress as much as an external stimulus can. When we feel empty or lacking, we slip into a limitation mindset where we can feel unworthy and demotivated. We can look to the external world and feel like a failure, developing feelings of not being enough, imposter syndrome or loneliness.

This 'hole' that generates stress can often be invisible (a void, a lack) at the start and if untreated or unaddressed it can become very visible as it impacts the physical structures and chemical messengers and hormones in our bodies. This can lead to stress-related physical ailments and a fracture in our mental wellbeing. Low mood and depression can often be the end products of a chronically dysregulated nervous system.

Stress can also show up as a result of the growth of thoughts and beliefs that were planted as seeds in your early life, often before the age of seven. Over time, these behaviours and beliefs germinate in your subconscious mind and form shoots, thorns and vines in your adult life. The self-limiting or

33

self-destructive internal narratives that were shaped and created in your early life generate habits in your later life that might not be the most beneficial to your nervous system. However, because you learned them growing up, they became the norm. So breaking into a new thought pattern or cultivating a more positive or optimistic outlook can seem alien, wrong, scary, and push you completely outside your comfort zone. For example, perhaps you grew up in a world where people demanded a lot from you: you had to be the grade-A student, the best on the football team, the star of your school play, the 'good girl' or the 'good boy'. So now, in adulthood, perfectionism plays out strongly. You hold yourself to too high a standard and place too much pressure on yourself. This, in time, leads to huge cracks and strains in your life: the constant pressures, the never-ending to-do lists, always feeling under-accomplished, and the constant busyness that often results in burnout.

It's important to understand that the body reacts to both *actual* stress and *perceived* stress in the same way. Our nervous system cannot decipher whether we are experiencing an actual threat or a perceived threat, meaning that if we *think* there might be danger ahead, even if that danger never manifests, it will activate the nervous system and our stress response. This is why the power of our thoughts is so incredible when it comes to whether our nervous system is regulated or dysregulated.

Through greater internal awareness, we can begin to manage our stress that little bit better. With various lifestyle tweaks, we can steady the ship. And once the ship is steadied, no matter what storms we face, no matter how big the waves or how rough the seas, we can face it head-on with greater clarity, ease, centredness and perspective.

Our outer reality is like a projection of our inner thoughts, feelings and beliefs. The body is like the channel that transcribes the language of our nervous system through our reactions and responses, displaying them for the world to see.

Activating the vagus nerve

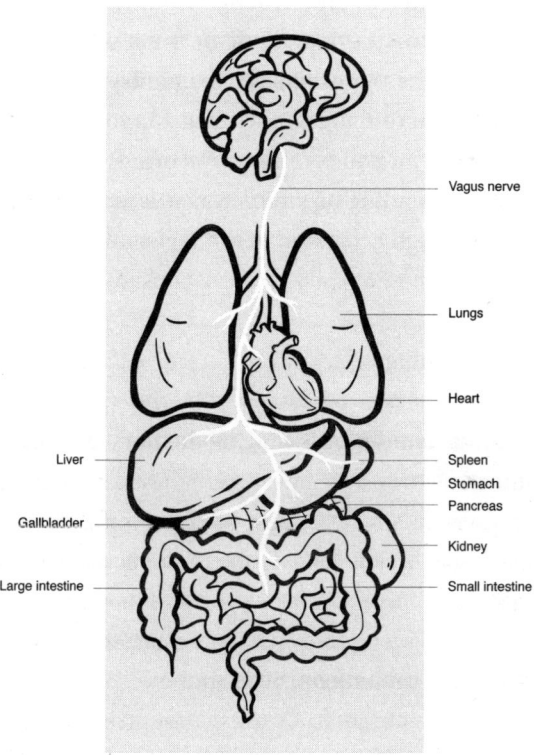

The vagus nerve, also known as the wandering nerve, is one of the longest nerves on the parasympathetic side of the nervous system. The vagus nerve takes a long, winding course through your body, starting from the part of the brain called the medulla, then branching down both sides of your throat, connecting with your tongue, heart, lungs, abdomen and digestive organs. In other words, it's a communication channel that runs between the gut and the brain.

Because it has such a wide reach, the vagus nerve allows the main organs of the body to communicate; hence it's responsible for the way your body reacts to stress. Likewise, when it's stimulated, your vagus nerve can move your body from a state of stress to a state of relaxation.

For greater health and healing, we want to move out of living in a dominant sympathetic nervous state and switch more easily to the opposite side, the parasympathetic side, which is all about rest, digest and repair. As you will see, there are many simple methods to move out of a dominant sympathetic state, depending on which way you react to stress, but one way is through activation of the vagus nerve. You can do this by:

* Deep breathing

* Practising mindfulness and meditation, even for a few minutes

* Engaging in breath-focused exercise, such as yoga, tai chi or qigong

* Listening to calming music or sounds

* Massaging the outside part of the ear, which contains a branch of the vagus nerve

* Spending time in nature

* Humming your favourite song, chanting or singing

* Cold-water immersion

* Having a good belly laugh

* Fascial manoeuvres and releases. Fascial manoeuvres involve movements or exercises that target the fascia, which is the connective tissue that surrounds muscles, organ, and other structures in the body. A simple example includes gentle neck stretches. This involves gently tilting your head to one side, bringing your ear towards your shoulder until you feel a gentle stretch along the side of your neck. Hold the stretch for a few seconds and then switch sides and repeat. This stretch can help release tension in the neck muscles and fascia, which can contribute to vagus nerve activation and promote relaxation and stress relief.

How do you respond to stress?

We are all different and we all react to stress – or perceived stress – differently. Our nervous system responds in different ways depending on our upbringing, thoughts, experiences and trauma, which have all marinated over time into subconscious programs that make us who we are.

Your body might roar and shout at you to put up your fists and fight; or it might urge you to avoid confrontation and flee. These are the well-known 'fight' or 'flight' responses. But your body might also warn you to 'freeze' – where you are unable to move, become numb; or push you into a 'fawn' state – where you try to please or appease. It might cause you to 'flop' – physically collapse or even faint – or you might find yourself moving into a flow state, where you are alert but at ease.

The six Fs are:

∗   Fight
∗   Flight
∗   Freeze
∗   Fawn
∗   Flop
∗   Flow.

Now I want to ask you a question. Which of these Fs do you default to as a form of protection or as a coping mechanism? The most common stress responses tend to be fight, flee, freeze or fawn. However, in extreme cases, you might flop; when you are aligned and centred, you might find yourself in flow. There is no right or wrong way to react; my question is simply a healthy 'poke' to stir up curiosity about your natural reaction when faced with stress.

You'll meet simple breathwork techniques and practices again and again in this book, because no matter what state you're in, using the breath as a gateway out of stress is incredibly powerful. Breathwork can be a great place to start to help regulate your nervous system. I believe it is one of the most important tools we have to help calm and rebalance our mind, body and soul. This is why you will find breathwork mentioned often throughout the book. If you would like more detail about why breathwork is important, go to page 272 in the Soul section.

Let's look at each of the F reactions a little further and perhaps you will recognise your default response.

Fight

When you are in a fight response, you might feel a sudden surge of adrenaline and a sense of increased energy, your heart rate might accelerate, your muscles might tense up and you might feel more alert. In this state, you could be prone to react in a defensive or aggressive manner, ready to confront the perceived threat head-on. Your body is primed for action and you might exhibit physical signs of readiness for action, such as a tense posture, clenched fists and focused eye contact.

However, on the inside, you might be experiencing something quite different. You could be feeling a surge of intense emotions, such as fear, shame, anger, frustration, embarrassment or anxiety.

Overall, as your nervous system navigates a fight response, you might feel a combination of emotional intensity, physical readiness and a mental focus. Does that sound like you or someone you know?

From fight to freedom

The good news is that it is possible to mobilise ourselves from a fight response to a state of freedom. We can coax our nervous system back to a state of regulation by taking some simple actions.

* **Use your voice:** Shouting, or even screaming, in a safe space, ideally where no one can hear you (for example into a pillow) can provide a release of built-up tension, stress and emotions. Vocal expression can release physical energy in the body and discharge excess adrenaline and cortisol. It's a way to vocalise emotions that might be difficult to articulate in words and provide a sense of validation and acknowledgement of those feelings, which can help in processing and coping with stress. (Please note, screaming at another person is *not* recommended.)

* **Physical action:** Punching a pillow or a punch bag, shaking out your body, going for a run or a brisk walk,

even stamping and sighing, shaking and twisting or contracting and extending your body can shake you out of a fight response.

* **Breathing:** Deep breathing is a powerful way to take us out of the fight response, when we might be breathing rapidly and shallowly from the lungs. The very act of deep, slow diaphragmatic breathing sends a signal to your body that you are safe. The body knows that if you are able to stop, pause and take slow, deep belly breaths you can't be in any danger. This switches on the parasympathetic side of the nervous system, allowing you to rest, repair, heal and digest. Finding a quiet place to centre and do these breathing techniques can be really helpful during stressful situations, for example, if you've just had a difficult conversation or a stressful day at work.

Breathing techniques

The following are some examples of deep breathing to help mobilise out of the fight response.

* **Lion's breath:** A powerful breathing exercise to help release tension, reduce stress and promote feelings of liberation and empowerment.
  » To perform this breath, inhale deeply through your nose, then open your mouth wide, stick out your tongue and exhale forcefully with a 'ha' sound. As you exhale, also make sure to open your eyes wide and gaze upwards towards your third eye (the space between your eyebrows). Repeat a few times to help release, recharge and regulate.

* **Letting-go breath:** This can help release tension, stress and negative emotions from the body and mind.

» Find a comfortable position. Close your eyes or lower your gaze. Go within. Inhale deeply through your nose, letting your belly rise. Hold the breath for a moment at the top of the inhale. As you exhale through your mouth, imagine releasing any tension, stress or negative emotions from your body and mind. Visualise these feelings leaving your body with each exhale. You can also use affirmations, for example *I breathe in spaciousness and light* (breathing in); *I let go and surrender* (breathing out); or *I trust in life* (breathing in); *I surrender my fears* (breathing out).

* **The cooling breath:** This helps activate the parasympathetic side of the nervous system.

» To perform this breathwork practice, curl your tongue into a U shape or slightly part your lips. Inhale slowly through your mouth, feeling the cool air passing over your tongue or lips. Close your mouth and exhale through your nose. Repeat this cycle for several rounds.

Self-talk and positive affirmations

We often default to a reactive fight response when we are triggered by stress. This is due to our locked-in subconscious programs. In order to change our subconscious programs and mobilise out of a fight response, we must be willing to not only *think* differently but also to *act* differently.

Negative thoughts and beliefs can contribute to feelings of anger and frustration. Practising positive self-talk by reframing and rephrasing what our inner voice says is a powerful yet simple way of shifting away from stress and promoting a greater sense of calm. We will discuss this in greater detail in the Mind section.

Flight

When I experience stressful or challenging times, my natural tendency is to retreat, throw the towel in and hide under my duvet. My default setting is to reject myself and my abilities and just hide away from the world. This is, of course, the flight mode of the sympathetic nervous system reaction.

The flight response can manifest as feelings of fear, anxiety, overthinking, worry or panic. Like the fight response, it is essential for survival in dangerous situations, but it can also be triggered by stressors that are not necessarily life-threatening, for example a deadline or answering a million emails or WhatsApp messages. The thought of these things drives up my blood pressure, creates tension, stress and strain in my muscles, gives me a feeling of havoc and urgency, and makes me want to shut everything off and run away.

I regularly use complementary therapies like acupuncture and reflexology for my wellbeing. During a typical session my therapist examines my body – and the body never lies. **Your body is a printout of what's going on in your mind and soul. The body simply shows us what the mind hears and what the soul feels.**

One day, she told me to turn over on my front, and she began working on my back. She began pushing on the various pressure points and acupuncture points. When she came to the area on my back that is linked and connected to my stomach, I nearly jumped off the bed with pain. Oh my god, that pain. She explained that this area is my stomach, and in Chinese medicine the stomach is associated with worry, overthinking and anxiety. 'Miriam,' she said, 'you are over-thinking, you need to slow your mind down.' These words resonated with me, as the racing busyness of my mind was now not just 'in my mind,' but was actually showing up physically in my body, which, of course, was impacting my digestion. This reinforced the impact of the mind–body connection and how stress and everything we think about impacts our physical health and wellbeing.

From flight to freedom
Write lists
When we're in flight mode we have a tendency to flee, which often leads to tasks not getting fully completed or only being half done. Writing lists and getting organised can help reduce feelings of overwhelm and stress. It can make you feel more in control of your daily tasks by helping you prioritise your needs, breaking your duties down into more manageable bite-sized steps. This can ultimately help you switch out of the flight response of the nervous system.

Stop pottering
We can spend our lives pottering, but what are we actually pottering for? It's a form of escapism – you keep yourself busy to distract from just being. When we remove the distraction of pottering, it can sometimes be uncomfortable or scary. If you have spent your life in flight mode, anxious, busy and pottering all the time, then stopping, stalling or slowing down can be quite frightening. This is because when we slow down and stop, the noise from within bubbles to the surface and we actually get to hear our inner thoughts and feel our inner whispers.

So, we must ask ourselves, what are we pottering for and does it make a difference? The other day, I caught myself in the kitchen pottering between the fridge and the sink and the kitchen table, putting things away, wiping down the counter, folding clothes, when I heard my little boy call me. He was playing in the playroom with his pirate ship and he called out, 'Mommy, Mommy ... can you come play with me, please?'

43

This halted me in my tracks. Ten years from now, will I remember what I was pottering for? Absolutely not. But will I remember going into the playroom, sitting on the floor and playing pirates with my son? Absolutely yes. That memory will be locked in my heart for ever; but pottering will always just be pottering!

Of course, housework needs to be done and dinner needs to be cooked, but not 24/7. Stop pottering and take a genuine break. When you're having your cup of tea, sit down and actually have it; when you're having your breakfast, lunch or dinner, sit down and eat it without distraction, without simultaneously sending emails, answering text messages or signing your kids up for activities! If you stay in that present moment and just be, you remove the distraction and free yourself from a constant state of flight. This can begin to break the cycle of staying stuck in a reactive stress state which only attracts more things to be stressed about.

The salvation of slow

For me, being in a flight phase is like being the Tasmanian Devil cartoon character – I am constantly spinning like a tornado, going, going, going. In this state of flight, your energy can be described as fragmented, frantic and frenzied, making it difficult to focus or concentrate. You might also have a sense of panic or overwhelming fear pushing you to take drastic action to escape a perceived threat. After intense periods of heightened activity, the nervous system can become overwhelmed, leaving you feeling exhausted, drained and emotionally spent. This is a hard type of energy to be around, but it's also a hard energy to live in. We are not always aware that we are walking around as this ball of chaotic energy. If you are in this energy right now, you are most likely fuelling yourself with caffeine and sugar to keep the frantic energy alive. You might not be able to think clearly, and you could be sweating or biting your nails. This energy has to go somewhere, so if you find yourself in this flight mode of constantly moving, doing, picking, pottering, try to move that energy out of your body in healthy ways such as walking, running, yoga, cycling, dancing. Once the emotion has been moved out in a healthy way, we must break the cycle and become more present by pausing, being, and slowing down.

Find your ground

Grounding is a wonderful way to bring you back into your centre and disrupt the fleeing tendencies. Grounding involves taking your shoes and socks off and earthing yourself, perhaps by walking on grass, placing your feet in the ocean, or pressing your feet into sand or the clay beneath you.

Physical activity and inner light activation

Engaging in movement and breathwork that bring fire back into your belly, raise your inner light and confidence, strengthen your solar plexus chakra (an energy centre located around the navel that is associated with inner strength, courage and confidence), and allow you to regain courage and hope is key to mobilising out of the flight response. For me, yoga and boxing were gamechangers. Sun salutations and core work really helped bring energy back into my solar plexus, while boxing greatly raised my 'yang' energy, strengthening my inner fire, enabling me to stand up for myself more, to back myself and find my strength, to challenge my inner stories and enable me to transcend from victimhood to victory. My inner strength is a muscle that I am still assembling, but I am loving the challenge and enjoying the revealing process.

Freeze

The freeze response is another coping mechanism when responding to a stressful situation and is one that I see a lot of clients getting stuck in. The freeze response leaves one temporarily paralysed by fear and unable to move. In this response, rather than fighting off the danger or running away from it, we do nothing. We freeze.

A good example of a freeze response is when someone experiences 'stage fright' – they may forget their lines or even be unable to perform.

It can be described as 'attentive immobility'. While the person who is 'frozen' is extremely alert, they are also unable to move, resulting in what we call 'tonic immobility'.

Think of it like driving a car. When you're in fight mode, you're putting the foot to the floor and accelerating really fast. When you're in flight mode, you're braking. When you go into freeze mode, you hit the accelerator and the brake at the same time, which results in the car stopping, or freezing.

Freezing as a response to a threat might seem effective, a sort of 'playing dead' in the face of danger. Consider an animal being attacked by a predator – if the animal freezes, plays dead, the predator might leave it alone. And so this freezing response plays a valuable role in providing protection in the face of danger. It might be effective temporarily, but it's ineffective in the long term, as it can manifest as an inability to communicate, react or take any action of self-preservation, thus eroding our sense of self-belief and inner strength.

It's important to note that being frozen is not a collapsing or a letting go. Collapsing (the flop response) occurs when the muscles literally flop and your whole system drops and falls. Freezing, however, is where there is tone in the body, but there's no movement.

How does it work?

Dropping into a frozen response often occurs when you perceive that you can't fight the danger or stress, because you simply don't have enough energy to attack or you feel that fighting would be ineffective. Yet you feel that you can't flee from it either; you can't run because you just don't know where to go. So you become numb. Why? We freeze so we don't have to feel. **When the attachment to flight and the defensiveness of fight are at odds with each other, you go into a freeze zone.**

A freeze state can manifest itself in many ways, but the most common are:

Procrastination

When we procrastinate, we freeze. The mind keeps going a million miles an hour, but our actions are halted. Nothing gets done, yet the noise in our mind gets louder and louder, and this results in a numbing out to avoid the reality of the uncomfortable emotions we are perceiving, most commonly fear, judgement, ridicule, not feeling good enough, imposter syndrome and shame.

Have you ever had a big exam coming up, and you knew how important it was for you to study, but perhaps you were dreading the exam so much that you couldn't bring yourself to do it? I found myself in a similar situation writing this book. I spent months and months putting it off, finding all the reasons in the world not to start, because beneath the surface, at the root, I was afraid to. Why? Because I was afraid it would be useless, that people would judge it and not approve of it, that I wouldn't have the capacity to write and that I would be ridiculed for it being a failure.

Procrastination also serves as a 'getting you off the hook' mentality, because by not writing the book, studying for the exam, applying for that job or asking your crush out on a date, it prevents the pain of rejection – the shame of not being approved of, accepted or respected.

Detachment or dissociation from trauma

If you experience grief or bereavement, yet you don't express a reaction or response to it, you can become numb. Some people delay processing or feeling the pain of a deep loss. You might see the partner of a loved one at a funeral and there's no expression of sadness or pain; they are emotionless. This is not wrong or 'bad', it is a normal reaction – the person simply can't go there right now. To feel the pain would be too much, so they shut off, dissociate and detach from the trauma until their nervous system is ready to face it and deal with it.

Inability to feel joy

There might be amazing things happening in your life but when you're in an overwhelmed state, and you enter the freeze zone, you simply can't feel light, love or joy. Physiologically and chemically, your hormone levels have been altered as a result of prolonged exposure to stress. The constant flooding of stress hormones impacts your gut, your brain and the secretion of your serotonin 5-HT (a.k.a. your 'happy hormone'). You might be living the most amazing life, but when your serotonin levels are low, you can't appreciate any of it. You're powerless. You're numb. You might be unable to feel the love that someone is showing you, or perhaps you are unable to celebrate your successes. There's a dimming down of your light, your brilliance and your beauty.

Body tightness, stiffness or heaviness

The muscles in your body might feel locked, trapped, tight, tense and frozen. It's as if your whole body has solidified into an ice cube and you've frozen, leading to rigidity. This rigidity in the body stems from the nervous system being overactivated and from an inflexibility in our way of thinking. Being rigid in our thoughts can result in this constricted energy sweeping through the body, creating tautness and tension. How many of us have ever felt stressed and, as a result, experienced stiffness in the neck, jaw, shoulders and lower back? Even if you haven't been doing any strenuous exercise, you experience pain and strain. This is because the mind has been tense, and overexertion in the mind will manifest as overexertion in the body. The muscles pick up on these signals and go into shutdown mode. When our nervous system is overloaded, the hormones of stress cause our musculoskeletal system to brace for danger. We see this predominantly in the fight response, but over time or with too much fighting, we can transfer over to a freeze response and so the body and its muscles can also feel frozen and locked.

Inability to express your needs

This is when you don't speak up or don't voice how you're feeling. Have you ever felt strongly about something, but you felt a restriction in your throat and you were literally unable to get the words out? In this situation, a freezing of your vocal cords occurs and you're unable to express how you feel or what you need. This differs from when you're in a fight response, when you might roar and shout. If you're in a flight response, you tend to go within, but still might express your anxiety, share your sense of overwhelm, your feelings of being scared and lonely. However, when you're in a freeze response, there is a lack of expression; there's a silence that can be deafening to the observer. Perhaps you want to scream but you simply can't – your vocal cords are frozen, unable to vibrate and release what you feel in your heart. This freezing occurs due to a threat or a fear that if you did speak up, you would be seen as foolish, stupid, wrong or bad.

From freeze to freedom

With any trauma or challenging situation, the hardest thing to do is to feel it in that moment. If freezing is how you have responded to a situation and you are now willing to come out of survival mode, you first have to thaw. **You have to melt all the numbness. This thawing process is where the melting ignites the feelings and the feelings ignite the healing.** This is the painful part, it's the hard work, but it is also where the dissolving away of fears and pains begins. You know when you've been out in really cold weather and your hands get so cold that you can't feel them, but when you heat them up under a warm tap, they start to sting before they feel better? That's like the thawing process. Coming out of a freeze response stings before you feel the warmth.

The great thing about being aware of the freeze response and being able to catch yourself when you're in it is that you can navigate your way out of it each time with more ease and grace, more awareness and confidence, and with a greater level of trust. I know this journey only too well, as I have experienced it on many levels. As a result, I have found freedom in many areas of my life where I was once completely frozen, so I'm passionate about sharing these learnings and practices with you so that you can find your way to freedom too.

In order to embark on this journey, you must first know that it is not always easy, it's not a quick fix and there will be tears. Without doing the work and feeling into the body, its sensations and its emotions, you will not be free. **In order to find spaciousness, lightness and freedom, you have to unclasp yourself from the prison of emotional pain.** The thawing process can be difficult, confronting and challenging.

It involves meeting parts of yourself that you don't want to meet. This 'meeting' will call for you to stew in uncomfortable emotions and sensations. You will find that it gets harder before it gets better. This is because in order to change, grow or evolve, an unravelling must first take place, a dissolving away of the old (old lifestyle habits and patterns, old self-negating beliefs, old unloving internal narratives and stories) so that a new way of living can emerge.

We can find ourselves in this place many times: it might be associated with our relationships, our career or our environment. It might happen as we navigate into a new role or identity, such as parenthood or loss. **Wherever and whenever the doors of life are revolving, opening or closing, the journey out of survival mode can be expected.** This journey can be beautiful, liberating and glorious. But it does take work.

Rule by A

I believe the first step to any change is to use my 'Rule by A' mantra:

* Awareness
* Acknowledgement
* Acceptance
* Action
* Achievement.

You must first have a healthy level of **awareness** that you are living in the freeze response. After awareness comes **acknowledgement**. *Can I recognise it? Can I acknowledge why I am here?* After acknowledgement comes **acceptance**. *Can I accept it right now, without judgement and without over-analysing?* There must be a healthy level of acceptance, an understanding of where you are, while understanding that it's not where you're going to be for ever. Then comes **action**. What are the key practical tips and tools you can put into action to mobilise out of freeze? And finally, how can I **achieve** freedom through the integration and application of these processes?

The first few steps can be quite challenging, because there tend to be a lot of suppressed feelings of overwhelm rippling from the soul, through the mind and into the body that triggered the freeze response in the first place. But it is possible if you stick with it. Trust that you will make it through those first challenging steps so you can find your way to action and, ultimately, a lighter, more content sense of self.

It's important to remember that you can't *think* your way out of a freeze response: you have to *do* your way out. This is because, as mentioned earlier, the prefrontal cortex (the area responsible for logical thinking) gets shut down in a stress response or a trauma situation, and the limbic part of the brain (survival mode) will fire up. This is why when someone's in a chronic freeze state, you can't simply tell them to come out of it, you have to help them to physically 'do the work', daily, regularly and consistently.

Here are some practical tools, tips and guides to mobilise out of a freeze state.

Re-engage the body

If you've been locked in a freeze response, your body will physically feel like a solid block: tight, tense, hard, with very little tone or flexibility. So a good way to thaw is to engage and move the body. This must be done in a delicate way that won't over-ignite or stimulate the nervous system too much. This technique is often used by therapists, who get patients to wiggle their fingers and toes or stamp their feet on the ground.

Other simple yet powerful methods are:

* Tapping the body (see page 90).

* Progressive muscle relaxation. You can do this by sitting or lying down, focusing on tensing one muscle group (like your hands or shoulders) for a few seconds and then releasing the tension while paying attention to the sensation of relaxation. Repeat this process for each muscle group, moving from head to toe, and remember to breathe deeply.

* Wrapping your arms around your torso and giving yourself a big hug.

* Gentle stretching.

* Neck rolls.

* Yoga, Pilates, qigong or tai chi.

These can all subtly bring awareness back into the body, helping you move out trapped emotion and suppressed thought responses. Mobilising the body brings healthy energy and flow back into your life.

Smells

Using soothing smells, such as incense, candles or essential oils, is a wonderful way to bring yourself back into your body as they can send signals to the limbic system to relax the body and mind, reducing the freeze response. Scents have been used for years in most religions and healing spaces; for example, you might smell incense when you enter a church or when you go to a spa. I use essential oils to help anchor and ground me before my keynote speaking engagements as well as in all my meditation workshops and yoga classes on our Soul Space retreats. They help calm and centre me, as well as the group.

Some examples of soothing or calming essential oils are lavender, chamomile, bergamot, rose, ylang-ylang and frankincense.

Breath

Breathwork is probably the most important way to refuel the body with energy and flow and instigate the thawing process. Start taking some slow, deep belly breaths. Again, this engages movement in the body, because the belly is rising and falling with each breath. With breathing practices, you are moving stress out and anchoring yourself back into your body.

Certain breathing patterns can be used specifically to mobilise out of freeze. You must be careful with what breathwork practices you use because some can aggravate or intensify the response if you are in a fragile or vulnerable position. Many of the breathing techniques that come from yoga have a wide range of health benefits in this thawing process, but not all breathwork practices are suitable for people with trauma to undertake on their own. Things that can aggrevate trauma include aggressive breathwork like holotropic breathing or breath holding. These can often mimic the stress response, which can aggravate and activate even more internal stress. This is why it is always necessary that these practices are done in the presence of a trained therapist, if you have trauma. While these practices might create an altered state of consciousness in people *without* trauma, they can be more damaging to a person who has trapped survival energy in their system. Slow, steady and subtle breathing is best.

* **Diaphragmatic breathing** (belly breathing) involves taking slow, deep breaths into the belly rather than shallow breaths into the chest. This type of breathing can activate the body's relaxation response and help to calm the nervous system.

* **Box breathing** is a relaxation and rhythmic breathing practice that involves taking slow, deep breaths in a pattern that creates a square or box shape. To do box breathing, firstly inhale slowly and deeply through your nose for a count of four seconds. Pause or hold at the top of the inhale for another count of four seconds. Next, exhale slowly and completely through your mouth for a count of four seconds. Finally, pause and hold your breath at the end of the exhale for another count of four seconds before starting the cycle again. Repeat for several rounds or for a few minutes to really reap the benefits.

* **Alternate nostril breathing:** This is a wonderful practice to help balance the nervous system and calm the mind. To do this, firstly find a comfortable position. Eyes can be opened or closed. Place your right hand (or dominant hand) in front of your face with your thumb and pointer finger forming a 'V' shape. Close your right nostril with your thumb and inhale through your left nostril. Let your pointer finger and middle finger rest on your third eye area (the space between your eyebrows). At the top of your inhale, bring your awareness to this third eye region, and relax. Then close your left nostril with your ring finger. Release your thumb and exhale through your right nostril. Again, pause at the end of your exhale and relax. Then inhale through your right nostril. Close it with your thumb. Release your ring finger and exhale

through your left nostril. Repeat several times, alternating nostrils.

It's important to remember that everyone's response to stress and threat is different, so it might take some experimentation to find the breathing exercises that work best for you. When in the freeze response, practise these techniques regularly to build resilience and regulate the nervous system to feel more ease, safety, harmony and alignment.

Meditation and mindfulness

Practising micro-meditative moments daily can have a profound impact when you are trying to move out of a chronic freeze zone. Start small: begin by engaging in 5–10 minutes of meditation or mindful practices (things that allow you to slow everything down and become more consciously aware), for example:

* **Sit mindfully** without distractions. Switch off your phone, remove external stimuli and simply breathe.

* **Eat mindfully:** No phones, TVs, laptops, books or newspapers at the table. Simply observe your meal. Take time to savour the smell, say grace, acknowledge where the food has come from, check in with how hungry you are, how full you are. Take time to chew your food, place your knife and fork down between each mouthful. Not only will this start to regulate your nervous system, it will also aid your digestion and help with weight loss, as we often inhale our meals without even noticing and fill ourselves up far beyond what we actually need.

* **Walk mindfully:** Take ten minutes to go for a walk and get some fresh air, and leave your phone behind. Slow down the pace of your walk, take time to notice your pace. Often the speed at which you walk can give insight into the speed at which your nervous system has been running – 'Speed often hides the need.' When we slow everything down, our needs, wishes, desires and home truths can bubble to the surface and be seen. When we feel seen, we feel more loved. When we feel more loved, we feel happier. When we feel happier, our nervous system will be more at ease.

* **Visualisation meditations:** Each morning, take a few moments to sit, be still and visualise being in a safe space. Visualise your body being safe, protected and grounded. Visualise yourself feeling aligned, strong, capable and beautiful. Visualise how you want to see yourself living in the day ahead. Visualise yourself being healthy, happy, organised, secure and harmonious. Your subconscious mind does not know the difference between the real and imaginary; it will just manifest whatever you feed it. The more you feed your subconscious mind with images and visions of what you want, the more you can manifest it in your life.

Life-serving affirmations

Affirmations are powerful ways of telling your subconscious mind that all is well. Try repeating the following to help you regulate your nervous system: *I am safe. I am capable, I am strong, I can do hard things. Today is a new day, a day where all is well and I am safe.* We will discuss this further in the Mind section.

Diet and nutrition

A balanced diet plays a crucial role in regulating the nervous system. The more processed food we eat, the more caffeine, sugars, alcohol and unnatural foods and beverages we consume, the more out of alignment and dysregulated we become. We'll take a deep dive into this later in the book (see Chapter 4).

Support

You have to have your people along the road – people you can talk to, who you can share your thoughts with, who you can trust. In order to move out of dysregulation, you must be willing to let yourself be vulnerable. If that sounds very scary for you, it means you have hit a resistance point, almost like when an acupuncturist or a massage therapist presses on an acupressure point and you jump off the bed with the pain! The pain is a just a symptom of a blockage or a build-up of pressure (usually an emotional build-up that manifests physically). If sharing your vulnerabilities sounds scary to you, please don't worry – you are not alone. Most people have parts of themselves that they want to keep hidden from the world. But the only way, I believe, that we can develop a more balanced nervous system and, therefore, greater mental, emotional and physical health is if we begin to unravel and speak through our vulnerabilities.

We have to remove the stigma that 'sensitive' means 'weak.' We have to be willing to put our hand up and say, 'Okay, I need to get mobile again, I need to move all of these emotions out.' It's like a cube of ice dissolving – if you leave it on the table, it's just going to melt and go everywhere. You need to put the cube in a glass so the water is contained, it's held. So what's your container? Who holds you? It might be a qualified therapist, a trusted friend or a family member. Your support might be from a peer group, class or community workshop you attend regularly. We all need a safe person we can go to when we start to dissolve so we can be held, heard, supported and seen.

Fawn

The fawn response is another survival mechanism. It involves complying after you've tried fight, flight or freeze several times without success. It is where one submits to or appeases others in order to avoid conflict or harm.

The fawn responses can be recognised in the following behaviours.

People-pleasing

This is a common stress response which involves constant appeasing, pacifying and trying to comfort people who threaten us. It acts as a soothing mechanism to avoid confrontation, prevent arguments, dispel anger and tension, and halt feelings of rejection or disapproval. The fear of not being accepted for being 'good', 'kind' or 'loving' is simply too much for your nervous system, so engaging in people-pleasing is a way of feeling part of the tribe. Feeling left out, left behind, rejected or abandoned are some of the greatest emotions that rattle our nervous system, so we learn to do whatever we can to fit in, including doing things that are against our core values.

I grew up with a built-in belief that if I was kind, loving, generous, lovable and likeable, I would be approved of, I would be accepted, I would be appeased. This led me to be a 'social butterfly'. In my teenage years, being known as 'Miriam the social butterfly' was something I was naively proud of. It meant that I was socially accepted (or so I thought) in many different groups. It meant I was liked, I was the centre of the party, and I loved this because it made me feel loved and approved of. This was everything for me. But as I grew and matured, I realised that always needing to be approved of led to many dysfunctional coping mechanisms in my life. It meant that I was like a chameleon, making myself fit into whatever group I became a part of. But if you are fitting into every group, you are not really being authentic or aligned with your true values. It means you can be swayed in many directions, pulled along with the crowd like a sheep, acting in ways that mirror the group that you are longing to belong to.

In one way, this had many benefits – it meant I had enormous fun and a sense of belonging – but it also came at a cost. It frazzled and frayed my nervous system, and this really came to a head in my twenties. I was living in Australia, and part of me was 'Miriam the social butterfly', the first one to the party, the last one to leave. This, of course, was part of my soul's calling – I love to have fun, I love to be adventurous, I love that free and passionate part of myself. However, I felt divided, because this part of me went far past the limits of my nervous system, and the reality was that there was another part of my soul that was screaming at me – the part that longed for solitude and silence and introspection. My spiritual self longed to go deeper in life, to transcend the materialistic world, beyond the surface conversations: 'How are you?' 'Yeah, fine.' Part of me wanted to rip all that open and delve into the more important conversations in life, the soulful conversations that carried depth and meaning. **I wanted to live a heart-centred life, not an ego, head-centred life.** This was bursting open within me, but I was so terrified of this part of myself that I had kept it hidden for many years.

I was in Sydney one day and, after a weekend of socialising and travelling, I went to a local park. As I sat there, I spotted a beautiful church in the distance. I was journalling in the park with the sun shining down on my teary-eyed face, asking myself some deep, open and honest questions. When I heard the church bell ring, I got up and went into the church. I sat in this beautiful space in silence, lit some candles, and I wept and prayed for guidance. I felt lost. I felt like there were two different Miriams and I didn't know which was the real one.

So I started to let out the part of myself that I had kept hidden – I like to call it 'coming out of the spiritual closet'. The world was different then, yoga was just becoming popular, spirituality or the 'wellness world' wasn't really a thing, so stepping into this arena was new for me and for many of my peers at the time. I started to travel all over Australia, soaking up everything I could in terms of holistic health, self-development, spiritual healing and health and wellbeing. I attended workshops by the Dalai Lama, I went to 'I can do it' conferences held by Hay House, which hosted the most incredible minds in the world of spirituality and self-development. I got to meet Louise Hay, Deepak Chopra, Marianne Williamson and more.

Then I went on to do many solo retreats across the country, and I spent weeks as a WWOOFer – a 'willing worker on organic farms'. I worked with families in the rainforest, I went on Angel Intuitive courses, detox retreats in Bali – you name it, I did it! This opened a gateway to my higher self and allowed me to go from living a divided life, where I felt as if there were two Miriams at loggerheads, to merging into one soulful, whole Miriam. I started to unravel some of the people-pleasing traits that had become destructive, and I began working with the most incredible psychotherapist who helped me through these blocks and barriers (and I still work with her to this day). I began asking why I was a people-pleaser in the first place. Was it because I feared that I was not enough as myself? As I started to remove the mask, remove

61

the need to be a certain way, it liberated my soul and allowed me to follow a path that was more authentic, aligned and peaceful.

Being a people-pleaser was a fawn response for me. I still have to be mindful of this, because I can default back to it if I'm off-centre, tired or overwhelmed, but having the awareness to catch myself when I go into this people-pleaser fawn response is one of the greatest gifts I have been able to give myself.

Lack of boundaries

Boundaries aren't always visible – yes, they can be physical, but they can also be emotional. Healthy boundaries are developed to create safety and security; however, if you are prone to people-pleasing and find yourself in a fawn state, it is likely that you have 'leaky' boundaries. You might let people into your energy space quite easily, appeasing them while denying your own desires and needs. You might think that people-pleasing is a kind thing to do, that you are being nice to everybody, but it can also be viewed as a manipulative way of living your life, because you are not living a life that's true.

We often don't create solid or defined boundaries for fear that we will be seen as stern or not kind, so we let people walk all over us, creating a whole world of messiness and stickiness. By doing this, we are actually manipulating other people to like us, because we are showing them only the side of us that we want them to see, which is not a true reflection of who we are.

Imagine a child cycling home in the dark. They come to a bridge. If there are no barriers on the bridge, the child will cross it with immense fear. But if the bridge has strong walls or 'boundaries', the child will fly across the bridge with no worries, no fear, no doubt. The walls of the bridge are similar to the boundaries we create in our lives. When we have clear boundaries, we feel secure – we know exactly where we stand because the boundaries create clarity and ease.

It might feel strange at first to create boundaries by saying 'no' and prioritising your own needs ahead of others'; it takes courage and patience. But the more we strengthen this muscle of creating healthy boundaries, the more we create ease in our lives and for those around us, helping us move from the fawn state and into a state of freedom.

How do you create more boundaries? It can be as simple as prioritising your values, learning to love and respect yourself and knowing that when your boundaries are stronger and more defined, you will have a less stressful life.

In effect, setting boundaries is like building a fence around your own personal garden. Just as a garden needs boundaries to keep out pests and weeds, you need boundaries to keep out negativity and unwanted burdens. It's important to say no to things that drain you and yes to things that support you. I give some practical examples on how you can create personal boundaries on page 113.

Over-explaining and over-apologising

As a self-labelled 'peacekeeper' and 'people-pleaser', the concept of over-explaining became my norm. Why? Because I needed to explain, justify and validate myself to the world. In terms of the fawn response, over-explaining occurs when we excessively justify or rationalise our actions or decisions in order to appease or please others. This behaviour often stems from a desire to avoid conflict or from a fear of rejection, leading us to provide more information than necessary in an attempt to gain approval or avoid negative consequences.

The root of a lot of over-explaining is that we don't value ourselves enough, so we have to explain, justify or please in order to be approved of, loved, seen or appreciated.

When you go into this fawn response of over-explaining, you are squeezing the nervous system. It gets revved up and agitated. As you enter that over-explaining state, you will often find that you speak faster or start fidgeting. The nervous system is not happy or at ease in this state, and the body processes this energy with bodily (somatic) expressions such as foot-tapping or shifting your weight from one foot to the other as you give a lengthy and detailed explanation of something. This physical restlessness might indicate that the person is feeling anxious or insecure, which is causing them to explain themselves excessively.

Not everybody is going to like everything you say or do, and being okay with that is the key to freedom and a regulated nervous system. We must remember that we're all different, and beautifully so. It's important to celebrate your uniqueness and the different choices you make. As long as they're true to you and true to your heart, you don't need to explain those choices to anyone.

From fawn to freedom

Moving from a fawn state to freedom involves a deep journey of self-discovery, healing and empowerment. It requires acknowledging past patterns of people-pleasing, setting boundaries and reclaiming your authentic voice.

Confidence

Greater self-worth, self-confidence and worthiness is key to moving out of a fawn state. Confidence is something that we can all nurture, develop and continue to work on throughout our lives.

One of the simple ways to do this is to begin with the things that you can control:

* **Start with your values.** Select three or four values that you would like to define you as a human being and then try to live those values every day. For example, you can make statements such as *I'm kind, I'm loving, I'm calm, I'm trustworthy*, etc. When you see yourself committing to and living those values consistently, your confidence will begin to rise. You get to control your values every day, and that can be a basis for your confidence to flourish.

* **Then examine your self-talk.** Every single word you use is either increasing your confidence or decreasing it. If someone gives you a compliment, just say thank you. If there is something you're not good at, just say 'I'm improving', 'I'm committing to getting better.' Make sure that your self-talk is the voice of your self-coach. Allow yourself to grow by making mistakes and forgive your mistakes quickly and easily. We won't get it right all the time and, as long as the inner voice is one of an inner coach, it will guide us to develop a sense of self-esteem, self-worth and self-confidence.

* **Finish with consistency.** After identifying and living your values, and paying attention to your inner voice, the final step is to develop the habit of consistency. Write down one or two things, no matter how simple, and do those things consistently. A person who always does exactly what they say they're going to do is generally a confident person, as their life is backed by an unshakeable truth in showing up and backing themselves. Consistency is an incredible way of building self-confidence because it provides faith and evidence to back yourself up, rather than the fear and uncertainty of self-doubt. Don't allow yourself to commit to something that you are not sure you

can deliver on. If you say you're going to do something, no matter how big or how small, be sure to execute it. That's how we build self-confidence.

Please also remember you are here for a reason: you have a story to tell, a mission to live, so stop playing small. Marianne Williamson's brilliant advice applies here: 'There is nothing enlightened about shrinking so that others won't feel insecure around you.' So step forward with joy and ease, with humility and confidence. Step into your power. Step into your truth. Begin small and build gradually.

Reflective visualisation exercise to cultivate greater self-confidence

An audio recording in which I guide you through this meditation can be found at www.soulspace.ie/lightup with the password LIGHTUP.

Close your eyes, take slow deep breaths in and out, bring your awareness to your third eye (the area between your eyebrows). Imagine a beam of light radiating out from this third eye centre, and in this light is a beautiful vision of you, as if you're watching yourself being projected onto a movie screen. See yourself radiating with self-assurance, poise and inner strength. What does this version of yourself look, sound and feel like? Picture yourself standing tall, gracious, self-assured and happy. Feel yourself embodying these elevated emotions of joy, strength and confidence. Feel your body being flooded with 'happy' chemicals such as endorphins and serotonin, changing your chemistry and biology and raising your frequency. Continue this practice for as long as you need.

Journalling

When you have finished this visualisation, ask yourself what daily practices you can include in your life to manifest this vision into reality. What do you need to stop doing, start doing or continue doing?

To emerge out of the fawn response, ask yourself questions such as:

* Is this something I really want to do in the deepest of my heart's desires or am I trying to meet someone else's expectations of me?

* Is this aligned to my core values?

* Do I have the energy and strength to commit to this?

* Would this bring me closer to feeling more ease and harmony and grace in my heart or would it bring me closer to feeling more struggle, strain and stress?

* Am I honouring my own needs in this situation or am I placing the needs of others before my own?

Boundaries

As discussed earlier, having 'leaky boundaries' can be a symptom of the fawn response, so take time to check in with yourself to see if you are saying 'yes' to something to appease others, especially if saying 'yes' is at the expense of your wellbeing or goes against your core values. Perhaps there is a specific person who triggers this people-pleasing response, so try to set healthy boundaries with them. Assert yourself and communicate your needs effectively from a place of love. **When we operate from a place of love we release ourselves**

from the chains of guilt that can sometimes appear when we start to say no.

Body scanning

This is a powerful way to help you move out of a fawn response. When you feel triggered into appeasing, pause, stop, scan the body. Where in the body do you feel this need? Tune into the body, tune into the heart, and ask yourself: *Is this really something I need? Is this something I have space for? Is this something that's aligned to my desires and my soul's passion?* Your body will communicate with you in a powerful yet subtle way.

If your answer is 'yes', your heart will open, your stomach will soften, your shoulders will drop, your breathing will become slow and deep, and your jaw, temples and forehead will relax.

If it's a 'no', you'll feel like your heart is contracting, your stomach will squeeze, your shoulders will tense, your breathing will become shallow, you'll feel a clenching around the chest and jaw, and your temples and forehead will tighten.

Taking time to tune into the language of the body and the nervous system is an effective way to tune into your needs and move away from a fawn or people-pleasing response. It allows you to come into your heart more, creating more peace and ease in your soul.

Flop

In a flop (collapse) trauma response, the body may shut down as a final defence mechanism. This can result in complete physical or mental unresponsiveness, blacking out and even fainting. Fainting in response to being paralysed by fear is caused when someone gets so overwhelmed by stress that their muscles become flaccid and loose, and they physically collapse.

The following lifestyle behaviours and feelings may indicate someone in a flop response: appearing disengaged; missing or skipping work, class or social engagements; expressing limited emotion; depression, anxiety or apathy.

Freeze and flop both involve the inability to move. However, from a biological perspective the flop response looks very different from freeze. Flop is where the parasympathetic state is dominant, which is usually associated with rest and repair, but this is such an extreme response that you become limp and completely inactive. A person experiencing this collapse response may feel disconnected from their body, exhibit decreased heart rate, blood pressure and body temperature, and will have a blank stare as they become less aware of their internal and external world.

From flop to freedom

To get help and mobilise out of a flop response, it is essential to prioritise self-care and seek support from trusted individuals or professionals. Seek a safe environment: move to a safe and comfortable space where you can feel secure and minimise further stressors.

Practise grounding exercises, such as deep breathing, mindfulness or focusing on your senses, to help reconnect with the present moment. And, most important, seek professional support. Talk to your doctor, therapist or mental health professional about your experience and emotions so that they can provide strategies to cope with and overcome this traumatic response.

Flow

Flow state is where there is a harmonious balance between the sympathetic and parasympathetic nervous systems.

This balance allows for an optimal level of arousal that enables individuals to perform at their best while feeling calm and relaxed.

In this state, we are both alert and relaxed, engaged but calm. Our cognitive functions are optimised, and we are able to respond consciously rather than reactively.

You'll notice that flow state creates a perfect balance between 'relaxation' and 'focus', which means when your body is in flow state, it can generate just enough arousal from the sympathetic system to focus, while simultaneously engaging your parasympathetic system so that you're feeling relaxed and restored.

This flow space is by far the most powerful force we can be in as it brings us into a state of coherence. It is in this flow state that we can best deal with the uncertainty and adversity of life.

Resetting is possible

Our body has an innate natural intelligence that is mesmerising and fascinating. It's our powerhouse that keeps us alive every day. How often do we stop to give thanks to our incredible bodies for all they do for us?

Deep within our core lies a wisdom, a knowledge and an ability to thrive and survive without explicit instructions. The brilliance of our bodies is why we have to ask those deeper questions about how we came into existence, how our internal ecosystem and nervous system automatically know what to do to keep us alive, how we are built with an internal navigational system whose sole function is to keep us in balance, in coherence, in harmony. When we are living in balance and in harmony, this incredible powerhouse of a nervous system is our best friend.

Consider, for example, a woman I did some work with. She was in a high-pressure work environment and constantly felt stressed due to deadlines, her perception of a demanding boss and long hours. As a result of these external triggers, she experienced a range of physical symptoms, including headaches, fatigue and digestive issues. Internally, her body was in a state of constant hyperarousal, with elevated levels of stress hormones circulating throughout her system. Over time, this led her to burnout, exhaustion and, ultimately, a decline in overall health and wellbeing. When I met her, she was broken, depleted and overwhelmed. After a number of sessions focusing on lifestyle medicine and reducing her stress, getting her back into rest, repair and recovery mode (through activating the parasympathetic side of the nervous system), she was able to regain clarity, alignment and balance – and she recovered beautifully. She no longer works in that job, as she realised you cannot heal in the very environment that made you sick in the first place. She made subtle yet powerful changes that enabled her to see her own light, power and confidence, and thus found her way back to feeling like herself by living a more wholesome and authentic life.

Another lady in her forties from our Soul Space community was experiencing chronic stress in her personal relationships, and thus was developing symptoms of anxiety and depression. The constant worry, fear and tension associated with interpersonal conflicts can take a toll on both the mind and body. Internally, this lady was experiencing persistent feelings of sadness, irritability and emotional numbness. In an attempt to escape the burdens and strains, she became over-reliant on drinking wine each night to take the edge off. This had caused knock-on effects, impacting her ability to think clearly the next day, making her feel tired and weary, and leading to a low motivation to exercise together with increased cravings for glucose-packed foods (i.e. sugary foods, caffeine and refined carbs) to keep her 'surviving' throughout the day. Over time, this led to a deterioration in not just her physical health but also her mental health. Subsequently, she went to her GP and was initially prescribed antidepressants. When I met her, she was confused, lost and overwhelmed. I gave her space to pause, stop and speak. I got her to reassess her life and identify the root cause of her problems. When she addressed the stresses in her relationships, through having the courage to ask hard questions of herself and engage in open and honest conversations, everything changed. Honest, open and meaningful conversations enabled the couple to gain greater understanding of one another's needs, desires and expectations, and ultimately paved the way for a much more meaningful and deeper relationship. Lifting the lid and exploring the truth of what they both needed enabled them to see each other's vulnerabilities and move forward with greater compassion, understanding, forgiveness, connection and grace. She slowly began to regain a sense of freedom in her life, and combined with small lifestyle changes in diet, mindset, movement and breathwork, she was able to turn her life around and didn't need the pills after all. Of course, some people do require the assistance of antidepressants, but in the case of this lady, lifestyle changes enabled her to regain balance and harmony. (You must consult your GP before you make any changes to your prescribed medication.)

Your stress management toolkit

While the six Fs are all different ways we react to stress, there are common methods we can use to shake ourselves out of these challenging states and into one of clarity and calmness.

This might be helpful if you're not sure which way you're reacting to stress, or if your nervous system is so dysregulated that you can't see the wood for the trees. Trying a few of the following techniques can give you much-needed space to think and they can act as a great first step on your journey toward inner peace and calm.

* Embrace a breath-focused restorative practice like yoga, qigong, tai chi or any exercise that is done more slowly and places a focus on the breath, for example walking, hiking or swimming. This will activate the parasympathetic nervous system (our system for rest, digest and repair), allowing our nervous system to recalibrate.

* Commit to regular diaphragmatic breathing. Take slow, deep belly breaths throughout the day. Inhale through your nose, allow your belly to rise up slowly, pause at the top of your inhalation (a point of stillness), then exhale, allowing your belly to fall as you release tension and stress. This can quickly shift you out of the sympathetic nervous system and into the parasympathetic nervous system. It costs nothing and it can be done anywhere.

* Develop morning and evening routines. How you set up your day and close it down has a huge impact on your progress and productivity. Start your day with love (meditation, prayer, yoga, breathing, journalling, fresh air, a healthy breakfast) and close it down with gratitude (more on this later; see page 253).

* Develop a self-care practice. Get out in nature and awaken your spiritual self. Make time for the things you love to do. Nourish yourself and practise self-compassion

and kindness. Explore your relationship with busyness and your perception of urgency and pressure. Use the mantra WIN – What's Important Now? Prioritise what really matters. Create healthy boundaries. Self-care is a necessity. If you are healthy, happy and have greater peace of mind in your life, those around you will also naturally benefit.

* Prioritise and delegate tasks to lessen the load. Make a list of tasks and prioritise them based on their level of importance.

* Cold-water immersion. Jumping into the sea is my therapy; it is my reset. When you plunge into cold water, you can't think of anything else – the worries, fears and overthinking dissipate and disappear. You avoid fast-forwarding to the future or revisiting the past. It anchors you in the here and now. It also brings that childlike sense of adventure into your soul. You feel alive, excited and fulfilled. If you cannot get into the sea, simply have a cold shower. Start small – at the end of your shower, turn it to cold and stand under the water for 15–30 seconds. Breathe slowly and deeply. This is not just physically beneficial, it's also almost like a purification process, clearing away any negative debris or stickiness from your energy. You could also simply splash cold water on your face or rub an ice cube down the sides of your neck, which stimulates the vagus nerve. **Please note:** regular cold-water immersion is extremely beneficial for regulating the nervous system if your window of tolerance is wide; however, if you are in a severe state of overwhelm or fight or flight this may not be the best solution. In this situation warm baths may be more soothing for the nervous

system. It's important that you listen to your body and know that at different stages and phases in your life you may require different forms of therapy and support.

* Seek support. Talk to a friend, family member, therapist or support group when you need help coping with stress.

* Exercise regularly. Physical activity can help reduce stress by releasing many powerful chemicals which boost mood (more on this in Chapter 2).

* Get enough sleep. Make sure you are getting enough quality sleep each night to help your body and mind recharge. (There's much more on the importance of sleep in Chapter 3.)

* Pay attention to your diet. Reduce caffeine, sugary drinks, alcohol and stimulants. These will rev up the nervous system and drive more anxiety and stress (more on this in Chapter 4).

* Practise things like meditation, visualisation, positive psychology, positive affirmations, mantras, prayer. These are all powerful ways of reducing stress and enabling us to better deal with challenging times. We'll delve into this in detail in Chapter 6.

Physical tension, emotional stress and mental fatigue all need to be moved out of the body. Movement unravels these strains and enables an awakening of inner and outer freedom of mind, body and soul.

CHAPTER 2

MOVEMENT AS MEDICINE AND AWAKENING YOUR INNER PHARMACY

Movement and exercise were always built into my psyche. Growing up in a sport-orientated home, movement was something that I felt deep in my bones. From an early age we were aware of the importance and brilliance of movement and exercise, not just for physical wellbeing, but for inspiring a sense of community and a sense of joy. As early as I can remember, my life revolved around some form of movement. My two sisters and I did Irish dancing regularly and it became part of our daily life. When we were younger, my family ran a B&B, and most mornings my sisters and I would dance for the guests. Even though some mornings we cursed our parents for making us get out of bed and dance, I now see the importance of morning movement to awaken the heart, body and mind, for shaking out stress, grogginess and worries and lighting you up.

Camogie, hockey and swimming became big parts of my formative years, and later in life yoga became my world. Every time I engaged in movement or exercise, I felt a sense of joy, a sense of freedom, a sense of liberation in my soul. It wasn't until later in life, after having two children, that movement became less and less a part of my daily ritual. I let stories and myths like *I'm too tired* or *I'm too busy* infect my mind, and as a result my body became more stagnant, my mood less uplifted and my mind more tired. I know now why I became quite anxious in that time: the build-up of energy was not being released or expelled from my body. Anxiety is often heightened energy with nowhere to go. I know that in the very depths of my bones I need movement to make my heart come alive and to clear my racing thoughts or dissolve the 'active' mind.

I do believe, however, that there is a time and space for rest, recuperation and recovery, which I will talk about in detail in the next chapter. Finding the delicate dance between movement and rest is paramount to a harmonious and balanced nervous system. It is important to note that not all movement has to be forceful or adrenaline-fuelled; movement can be peaceful, fluid and gentle. Both types of movement are necessary and important depending on what age or stage of life you are in.

We all have phases in our life when we need rest and repair. For me, having two children in succession along with full-time breastfeeding and many sleepless nights meant I faced depletion, and it would have been wrong of me to add high-intensity exercise to an already worn-out body. Knowing what exercise is important for your body at different phases and stages in your life is key. There will be a time when you run marathons or perhaps play high-level sport, but there will also be a time where your yoga mat and gentle breath-focused movement such as qigong, walking or stretching will be your go-to. As we move through this chapter, we will discuss the importance of the different types of movements, the science behind their relevance to health and why, no matter what age, stage, shape or size you are, movement is key to greater health, vitality and life-force energy.

The vast and varied benefits of exercise

For years, I had been caught up in the whirlwind of raising kids and being chained to their bedtime, which left me out of the loop for joining particular movement groups or clubs. However, a friend's frightening health diagnosis stopped me in my tracks and made me say 'Enough'. I needed to honour myself, my body and my exercise. This led me back to the GAA pitch, back to a community-led running club and back into the yoga studio. It was as if a part of me that had been dormant for a long time suddenly woke up, bursting with exhilaration and freedom.

I started to notice a shift in my headspace, and a new-found clarity and calmness followed. Exercise became my outlet for releasing pent-up emotions and stress, a way for me to find peace and balance.

When you think about the benefits of exercise and movement, you might go straight to the physical dimension; and it is effective for obvious things such as weight loss, body shape and size. However, it also greatly impacts our mental wellbeing – it is a powerful mood enhancer, helping to regulate our emotional wellbeing by expelling unwanted, stale or stagnant emotions from the body; and for our soul, it sends us into a beautiful flow-like state. It improves our health, quiets the mind, reduces stress and enhances the mind–body connection. These mind–body–soul benefits of movement include:

Physical:

*   Reduces the risk of chronic disease, in particular heart disease, stroke, diabetes and osteoporosis

*   Aids better sleep

*   Increases libido and sex life

*   Increases bone health, flexibility, balance and co-ordination.

Mental:

*   Acts as a mood enhancer (it is a natural antidepressant – more on this later)

*   Busts stress

*   Improves concentration, boosts learning and helps you think more clearly.

Emotional:

*   Releases trauma and difficult emotions (anger, frustration, irritation, sadness, victim mentality)

*   Releases stagnant energy from the body.

Spiritual:

*   Helps you find your zen by promoting a flow-like state

*   Encourages inner harmony and ease

*   Opens a gateway to the peace that resides within you.

The price of inactivity

*'It's not that exercise is an antidepressant,
it's that not exercising is a depressant.'*
David Bidler, President, Physiology First

I have noticed that many clients, as well as myself at times, face health and wellbeing issues due to a lack of exercise and from living a sedentary lifestyle. (A sedentary lifestyle is defined as not actively exercising for 30 minutes per day, three days in a row, for three months straight.)

Did you know that physical inactivity puts adults at greater risk of cardiovascular diseases such as heart attacks and strokes, type 2 diabetes, dementia and cancers such as breast and colon cancer?

It is a major risk factor for disease, with 50–60 per cent of the population affected (compared with 18 per cent affected by smoking, 30 per cent by bad cholesterol and 29 per cent by high blood pressure). Physical inactivity causes 11 per cent of premature mortality (5.3 million deaths worldwide compared with 5.1 million smoking-related deaths). Beyond the physical, it results in poorer mental health, lower energy levels and decreased overall quality of life.

Living a sedentary life acts as a depressive. The natural essence of our being is to move, to be in flow, to be mobile, to be flexible, to be free. Our modern lifestyles have made us rigid, fixed and sedentary. We move in straight lines, almost in a mechanical or robotic way. In contrast, animals hang from trees, they bounce, they jump, they sway, they move. We, too, are meant to move, jump, sway. If we look back to ancient times, life revolved around being outdoors. We didn't have to go to the gym to be fit. Life was constant movement: people worked on farms, they chopped wood, they carried water, they climbed trees to get fruit, they harrowed fields. Life revolved around moving in order to survive. Being outdoors in the natural world was the norm. Now we get up in the morning, sit at a table to have breakfast, sit in a car, train or bus to get to school or work, sit at a desk all day from the age of four or five (and if you're working in an office you might be sitting at a desk all day from 9:00 am to 6:00 pm), then you get in your car to drive home again. So much of our time is spent inside in a rigid, fixed position.We have lost the natural tendency to flow and dance and sway and bounce and swing.

Of course, exercise alone does not achieve this; we're meant to move together in packs and with people we love and trust. We need a sense of community and connectivity combined with other lifestyle pillars such as sleep and rest and nutrition, but on the whole, when we move our bodies, we can help prevent some mental disorders by promoting the positive neurotransmitters and chemicals naturally released by the body and that give us a sense of joy, ease, peace, passion and grace.

The pharmacy within: movement as an antidepressant

As a pharmacist, one of the most fascinating things I have found in recent times is that we have an internal pharmacy within our bodies, in our muscles. This powerful internal pharmacy can help us create more harmony, balance and greater well-being.

It can be helpful to understand the neurotransmitters and hormones at play when we exercise to see how a simple thing like movement involves a complex network of chemicals in the body.

Exercise activates your greatest pharmacy within by secreting vital chemical messengers that can help transform your physical, mental, emotional, physiological and spiritual sense of self. Imagine – you can elevate your overall health and vitality from the very act of moving!

Some of the key chemicals that are released during exercise are:

'Hope' molecules

When our muscles contract, they secrete chemicals into our bloodstream, and among these chemicals are myokines. These are small proteins that travel to the brain, cross over the blood–brain barrier and act as an antidepressant – this is why they're nicknamed 'hope' molecules. These hope molecules are literally manufacturing antidepressant molecules which can make you more resilient to stress and depression, and the only way to get them into your bloodstream so that they can travel to the brain is to contract your muscles. Your muscles are like your own inbuilt pharmacy. When you contract your muscles by doing things like walking, hiking, dancing, swimming and weightlifting, you're going to be dumping these hope molecules into your bloodstream.

I love the fact that they're called hope molecules because they do exactly what it says on the tin. They're creating hope; they're creating a sense of possibility. This is why, as I was growing up, I always felt more confident, courageous, inspired and hopeful after exercising. Now, years on, I understand the science behind it.

Endorphins

Endorphins are often referred to as 'feel-good hormones', and they are one of the key chemicals released when we exercise. The word 'endorphin' is short for 'endogenous morphine' – 'endogenous' refers to anything that is made within, and 'morphine', as we all know, is a powerful pain reliever. It gives a sense of ease, an almost floating, high feeling, and it removes pain. When we exercise, we often get this endorphin 'high', a feeling of bliss or euphoria – you've probably heard the term 'runner's high'. When we exercise, we are creating our own internal morphine and our own internal pain relief. By triggering the release of these endorphins, movement can help to alleviate stress and improve our mental wellbeing.

Dopamine

Dopamine is known for its role in the brain's reward system. It is often associated with feelings of pleasure, motivation and activation, and it plays a pivotal role in regulating our behaviour and our mood. Dopamine can help us to create a sense of accomplishment and satisfaction, a sense of pride, courage and passion, which can serve as a motivating tool to continue exercising regularly. This can give rise to feelings of success and achievement, which has a ripple effect by creating greater clarity, creativity and performance.

Serotonin

Serotonin, another powerful neurotransmitter, is often referred to as the 'happy hormone'. It is primarily known for regulating our mood, which is why exercise is seen as one of the world's best natural antidepressants.

As a pharmacist, I spent years dispensing antidepressants, mainly SSRIs (selective serotonin reuptake inhibitors). These antidepressants used to fly off the shelves. Over the years, I observed the increasing number of antidepressants that were being dispensed every day. They seemed to be on every second prescription, and often prescribed to young adults in their early twenties. I'm not saying that medication is not required in certain instances, but I feel it's really important to share the fact that we can create our own internal pharmacy and well of serotonin, the neurotransmitter that SSRIs target, by simply moving our bodies.

When we engage in physical activity, the production of serotonin can help promote feelings of happiness and joy, contributing to a sense of improved mental wellbeing and health.

Adrenaline

Adrenaline is another powerful hormone that is released in response to physical exertion and stress. Adrenaline came up a lot in the stress chapter, and it often gets a bad reputation as it's associated with too much fight or flight – a sympathetic-activated side of the nervous system. However, as already mentioned, stress is not all bad. We do need a healthy level of stress to feel motivated, encouraged and to get tasks done. Adrenaline helps to increase our heart rate, blood flow and energy levels, which can enhance our performance and endurance during workouts. By stimulating and triggering the release of adrenaline, exercise can improve our physical performance and boost our energy, making it easier to push through challenging workouts and achieve fitness goals. The key is to rest, repair and recover post-workout to prevent burnout and regain balance in the nervous system.

GABA

GABA (gamma-aminobutyric acid) is a neurotransmitter in the brain that is known for its calming and inhibitory effects on the nervous system. It helps the brain disengage from fight or flight, thereby reducing stress and anxiety and supporting relaxation and restful sleep. Regular physical activity has been shown to increase GABA levels in the brain, which can promote an enhanced sense of wellbeing.

Oxytocin

Oxytocin is a neurotransmitter often referred to as the 'love hormone', the 'snuggle hormone' or the 'bonding hormone'. It plays a crucial role in social bonding, trust, empathy, safety, security and feeling a sense of connection and community. Research shows that physical activity can trigger the release of oxytocin in the brain. Exercise-induced release of oxytocin can contribute to mood enhancement, stress reduction and improved social connections.

BDNF

BDNF (brain-derived neurotrophic factor) is a protein that plays a crucial role in supporting the growth and development of new neurons and synapses in the brain, so it is often referred to as 'brain fertiliser' or 'miracle grow'. It is believed to help learning, higher thinking and decision-making. Physical activity, especially aerobic exercise such as running, can stimulate the release of BDNF, which helps to enhance brain plasticity, learning and memory. This is why a good brainstorming activity in work is much better after exercise or a walk in nature post-lunch. Getting active in the middle of the day helps prevent that afternoon slump, which is why movement is key to better decision-making and higher performance in work and in life in general.

Movement and the release of waste products from the body

The medicine of sweating

Sweating is considered a natural way of cleansing the body: it is often associated with eliminating impurities, improving circulation and boosting the immune system. Incorporating sweating into your daily routine, through practices such as exercise, sauna therapy or hot baths, can help to support greater health and wellbeing.

The lymphatic system

Acting as a team of dedicated cleaners, the lymphatic system is responsible for ridding our bodies of waste or by-products of the metabolism. It collects these unwanted substances from our tissues and escorts them to the bloodstream for filtration and removal. Working hand in hand with the immune system, it produces and transports white blood cells, controls inflammation, distributes nutrients, and manages fluid levels. Unlike the circulatory system, the lymphatic system operates without a pump; therefore it is reliant solely on the body to move so that it can literally pump the fluid around the body. It needs internal pressure, muscle movements, heartbeats and respiration to propel the lymph through its vessels. If we are not moving, then it is difficult for the lymph to move, which can lead to a build-up of unwanted waste materials in the body, leading to congestion, which can become a breeding ground for viruses, bacteria and ill health.

The main factors that cause blockages in the lymphatic system include lack of exercise, poor diet, environmental toxins, trauma, infection and stress. This is why we must move regularly throughout the day.

The symptoms of a congested lymphatic system might not be obvious at first. They could be things you are just 'putting up with' or that could be caused by other factors in your lifestyle. However, if you are experiencing any of these symptoms, it would be worth seeing if movement and exercise make a positive change: bloating, brain fog, chronic sinus infections, fatigue, headaches, puffy or swollen ankles or hands, skin conditions like acne, dryness or rashes, swollen lymph nodes in your neck.

How to stimulate the lymphatic drainage system

* **Rebounding, trampolining, bouncing, jumping, skipping, hopping.** You only need to jump on a rebounder or a trampoline for about three to five minutes to benefit your lymphatic drainage system. The gentle bouncing motion helps activate the one-way valves in the lymphatic vessels. This activation promotes better lymph circulation and aids the removal of waste products from the body. Try this first thing in the morning – it will help support your immunity while also making you feel great from the inside out. Win–win!

* **Heel drops** can help stimulate lymphatic drainage by promoting movement and circulation in the lower body, aiding the removal of excess fluids and waste products from the tissues. Heel drops can be done standing or seated. I recommend standing heel drops first thing in the morning, as it is a wonderful way to get you out of your head, calm down any racing thoughts and land you back into your body, helping to regulate your nervous system. I recommend seated heel drops anytime throughout the day – while sitting at your desk, while watching TV, while on the bus, etc. They can be done anywhere and at any time and cost nothing. Simply lift your heels off the ground, rising up onto your toes, take a deep breath in as you rise up, and then as you exhale lower your heels back down onto the ground. For extra movement, you can also raise your arms as you inhale and lift onto your toes, and swing your arms back down by the side of your body while exhaling and lowering down onto your heels. This is a beautiful, fluid-like movement that allows flow into the lymphatic system and fluidity into your mind and your nervous system.

* **Qigong and yoga movements.** Twists, backbends and mini flows that link poses with breathwork to create internal pressure and muscle contractions support lymph movement and overall wellbeing. Examples include neck rolls, hip rotations, arm swings, leg swings, seated chair twists, cat–cow pose, downward dog, child's pose, legs against the wall.

* **Lymphatic drainage massage.** Movement by touch in the form of lymphatic drainage massage improves lymphatic drainage but also aids relaxation and stress relief. Always go to a trained, qualified practitioner. You can also help move and stimulate your own lymphatic system at home by tapping/pumping and massaging (towards the heart) the areas in the body where the lymph nodes are located (the subclavicle area just above the collarbone, the neck, armpits, chest, abdomen, groin and behind the knees).

Moving emotion out of the body

Movement is key to moving any unwanted stale or stagnant emotions from the body. The word emotion (e-motion) means *energy in motion*. All our emotions are energy and need to be moved out of the body in order to prevent a build-up of tension and tightness. Long-term unexpressed, undigested or repressed emotions can lead to an excess of stagnant energy in the body and over time can lead to physical ailments, symptoms and diseases. The more jarring emotions and feelings of hate we harbour within us, the more uneasy the soul becomes, and a restless soul will yield a disjointed and agitated mind; and an uneasy mind will send ripples into the nervous system, creating dysregulation in the body. All are connected. Movement is a powerful gateway to harmonising mind, body and soul and creating a union of peace within.

A powerful way of moving suppressed or trapped emotion out of the body is through the art of tapping.

Tapping

Tapping is a holistic healing technique that involves gently tapping on specific meridian points on the body to release emotional blockages and promote relaxation. This practice is deeply rooted in the principles of Traditional Chinese Medicine (TCM), which teaches us that emotions are stored in specific organs and, when unbalanced or stagnant, can manifest as physical or emotional symptoms. By activating the body's relaxation response through tapping with these ancient principles, individuals can cultivate both emotional and physical wellbeing through this mindful, integrative process.

Each organ in TCM is associated with certain emotions. For example:

* **The lungs – grief and sadness:** When I worked as a pharmacist, I observed a trend. At first I thought it was just a coincidence, but the longer I practised, the more I noticed this phenomenon. When somebody had just lost a loved one, it was common in the coming weeks or months for this person to present with a prescription for antibiotics for a chest infection. I became curious about this so I began to watch out for it and document it over the years. It was only later, when exploring integrative health, that I realised the connection the lungs have with grief and sadness. This is a clear example of how emotions can impact the body's organs.

* **The heart – joy and happiness:** The blood of the heart nourishes us not only physically but also emotionally and spiritually. Joy nourishes the heart, so when there's an imbalance of joy in our lives, it can be expressed as agitation and mania (too much), or depression (too little). When you get emotionally unbalanced, you might notice your chest becoming tight or heavy. You might feel anxious, introverted, sensitive, tender and uneasy.

* **The stomach and spleen – worry and overthinking:** the stomach and spleen are energetically linked to worry, overthinking and mental rumination. When these emotions become excessive, they can lead to tension in the midsection, digestive discomfort or a sense of being mentally overwhelmed or exhausted. You might notice sensations like nervousness, tightness in the gut or difficulty grounding your thoughts.

* **The liver – anger and frustration:** If there's suppressed anger or overactive anger, there can be some blocked energy around the liver. An excess of anger or repressed anger inhibits the liver's function, leading to further emotional imbalance and feelings of irritation, frustration, resentment or aggression. Imbalance in the liver system can manifest physically with headaches, waking up between one and three o'clock in the morning, and tension in the neck and shoulders.

* **The kidneys – fear and insecurity:** Obviously we can't banish fear from our lives, but we can pay attention to it and work through it consciously so it doesn't paralyse us. The kidneys are said to be the root of our constitutional strength – our batteries of life so to speak. Prolonged fear,

or sudden fright or shock, will damage the kidney system and deplete our reserves. Conversely, excessive fearfulness or a tendency to frighten easily are symptomatic of weakness in the kidney system.

By tapping on these areas and focusing on releasing the associated emotion, you can help to move stagnant energy and emotions out of the body. When tapping, breathe deeply and remember your intention is not just to make the emotion go away, it is to connect, to be present, to accept and feel, even if it's a feeling of irritation, fatigue, anxiety or sadness. Feel free to introduce a mantra (mind tool) or an affirmation such as *I feel you, I see you, I hear you, I've got you, I love you, I release you.* This practice helps to rewire the brain's response to the emotion and can lead to a shift in perspective and the release of emotional blockages.

As you move through this practice, don't overdo it, but be aware that by waking up this feeling you're going to release stress.

When you have finished, pause, be still, breathe and scan your body. See how you feel physically, mentally, emotionally and soulfully. If you practise this regularly, you'll notice that less emotion gets backed up or blocked up inside.

The tapping practice

*   Begin by standing up straight, feet hip-width apart. Start to breathe deeply and gently and bring your attention inside your body.

*   To tap, you're going to use either your fingertips, a fist or a cup-like shape with your hands. Spend about two or three minutes in each area to start. Go at your own pace and intensity.

* Tap at the midpoint of the chest, at the level of the nipples. This will help to open the chest and support heart and lung Qi – helping to release emotional suppression, overwhelm, heartache, grief and sadness. Stay tapping here for a few minutes whilst breathing deeply. As you begin to tap and awaken hidden or trapped emotions, you might begin to feel some sensations, like a tingling, as feelings bubble to the surface. Please don't run from these feelings or hide them away; if they are in your body, they have taken up residency for a reason. The more you neglect them, suppress them, stifle them, the more power they will have over you. The more suppression they feel, the more depression they breed. The more neglected they feel, the more havoc they create beneath the surface. Be willing to welcome whatever emotions arise. Sit with them and feel the relief of not having to run, escape or flee; instead, stay, sit and just be with whatever appears.

* Move over to left side of the upper abdomen, right below the ribcage, and begin to tap here with the pinky side of your fisted hands. Go at whatever pace or strength you need. (You don't have to tap too hard, just enough so you can feel the vibration inside your abdomen). Try to relax your muscles. Those racing thoughts might become more evident than you noticed before. Bringing your breath and awareness to your body brings energy in, helping any stuck energy to be released.

* Move your tapping down to the lower left side of the abdomen. The more you tap to the left side of the abdomen, the more you are stimulating the large intestine. The more you tap towards the centre of the body near the belly button, the more you are stimulating the

small intestine region. The intestines are related with your feeling of comfortable digestion and your overall energy levels. By tapping around the navel region you are also stimulating the solar plexus, which is your energy centre for stimulating inner courage, confidence and strength.

* Move your tapping over towards the lower right side of abdomen – again stimulating the large intestine.

* Move your tapping up to right side of the body, right underneath your ribcage area. This is the area that houses the liver (anger/frustration, resentment). Tap here and breathe deeply. Introduce the lion's breath if you need help to really release withheld anger.

* Then move down to the area below the belly button, near the bladder. As you tap here you may feel the sensation of having to go to the bathroom or you may feel some irritation, nervousness or discomfort here. This area is related to your first chakra, the energy centre for feelings of safety, security, connection, feeling grounded and centred. Tapping here grounds energy, calms fear and promotes feelings of safety.

* Lastly, tap lightly on the crown of your head using your fingertips. This helps to reconnect body, mind and spirit, releasing feelings of disconnection and opening up the channel to divine grace, love and light.

* Slowly stop your tapping. Take a deep breath and make some circular motions with your hands, massaging gently clockwise around your torso. You may feel some warmth,

some vibration or tingling. All of this is a good sign of energy and emotion moving.

It's important to remember that tapping is a complementary therapy and should not replace medical or psychological treatment. It can be a helpful movement tool in managing emotions and promoting self-awareness and healing.

What is the recommended amount of exercise?

We are all different, so there is no exact prescription for everyone. Ideally, however, the recommendation is at least 150 minutes of moderate-intensity aerobic exercise (vigorous enough to elevate heart rate and breathing, but still allowing for conversation, for example brisk walking, cycling, dancing) or 75 minutes of vigorous intensity aerobic exercise (exercise that causes a significant increase in heart rate and breathing, making it more difficult to hold a conversation, for example running, playing sports) per week. This can be spread out over several days and can also include strength training (weights, resistance bands or body weight) exercises at least two days a week.

Say goodbye to the excuses

Here are some of the regular reasons or barriers I often hear people say when it comes to exercise resistance.

I'm too busy, time is moving too fast, I can't seem to fit it in

I can definitely empathise with these reasons. As a mom with young kids, trying to fit in exercise can be a real juggling act! However, time is not moving fast. There are 168 hours in every week – this hasn't changed and will never change. What's changing is the busyness of our minds and the distractions in our lives. In order to succeed in life, we need to learn to prioritise what's important. We can all find 15 minutes to scroll on social media, yet we find it hard to find 15 minutes to do some yoga in the morning or go out for a little walk. If we were just to prioritise our time a little better, I'm sure we could squeeze in a few minutes every day to walk/stretch/move in some way. I don't even like using the phrase 'squeeze in,' as it suggests that you are squashing yourself or pressuring yourself into something, when movement ought to be something that doesn't squeeze you – quite the opposite, it should expand you, liberate you, give you a sense of space and calm your mind. **After exercising you feel on a high because you are riding the endorphin wave, you feel strong, capable and confident, and it awakens the lion or lioness within, breeding more courage and respect and reverence for life.** Your beating heart comes alive, your blood pumps with a sense of accomplishment and you begin to pulsate with energy and strength. Movement transcends the physical and enters the emotional realm and can be a catalyst for the soul to find purpose, meaning and passion. Movement is not something to squeeze or squash into your day; it deserves to be a non-negotiable, because its benefits are far too valuable when it comes to your health, immunity and wellbeing.

Remember, movement doesn't have to mean going to a gym and pounding it out. It can be as simple as playing with your kids, dancing around the room to your favourite song, gardening, taking the stairs instead of the lift or even window-shopping!

I'm too tired, I don't have the energy

If you are feeling tired all the time, it might be a result of your body being sluggish due to a lack of movement. If we don't move, we can feel stuck and lethargic. Exercise actually gives you energy. Next time you are on the couch feeling tired, challenge yourself to put the runners on, bring the dog for a walk, call a friend and get out for a stroll, do some simple stretching or even put on your favourite song and have a dance. I promise you you'll feel more energised and refreshed afterwards.

Even when every morsel of your being and your ego mind is screaming, *Noooo! I'm too tired, I don't want to do this*, instead of fighting the voice inside, lean into the resistance with compassion and say, *I hear you, thank you. But I am choosing not to play this tune right now*. Then drop out of your head and into your heart and let the ripples of love for yourself be heard. Let the heart encourage you to gently move in whatever way your body feels called to in that moment. It might poke you to run, walk, sway, dance, stretch – be guided by your heart, not your head, because your heart wants you to be healthy, happy, strong. Your heart wants you to be at your daughter or son's wedding twenty years from now; your heart wants you to be there for your grandchildren, to be at their school concerts, to be able to bring them to the park, to run around with them. Your heart wants you to be able to travel when you are eighty and live an adventurous life that is fuelled by mobility, flexibility and freedom and not ruled by pills, walkers or hospital visits. Yes, it can be hard sometimes to override the ego voice. Yes, it can be hard to get up and out on a wintery day. But it's also hard to be in chronic pain, to have chronic ill health and depression or low mood. You get to **choose your hard**. Which one do you want? This might sound harsh, but the reality is we have a lot more power and control over our future health than we think. The choices you make today will create your future, and by moving your body every day, you are creating a future of good health and vibrancy.

It's too hard, I'm not athletic enough, exercise just isn't for me

First, although it can be difficult, exercise should never be painful. It should challenge you and your muscles in a healthy way, but it should not be causing you pain. Movement should not be about punishing yourself. If you are finding yourself in this mentality, it is likely that you are approaching exercise from a place of fear which, in the long term, can be unhealthy and destructive. Instead, try changing your mindset, perspective and relationship with exercise. Seek out help from a trained professional or physiotherapist who can help you devise a safe and appropriate movement package specific to your needs and abilities. Instead of coming from a place of fear, try approaching movement from a place of love. Affirm to yourself, *I love and respect my body enough to move it and look after it.*

I'm too overweight/old, I'm not healthy enough to exercise

It's never, ever too late to start. Rome wasn't built in a day, so take small steps in the direction of your goals. For example, start by taking 15 minutes three times a day to do some form of movement, maybe stretching, walking or weights. Breaking it down into bite-sized, manageable chunks can make it more sustainable and enjoyable and help build consistency. You are enough and your body deserves to be healthy and happy. Be patient yet persistent, and remember to come from a place of love, not fear. Seek help and support and cherish your journey. You can do it. Small steps every day will go a long way. Your body wants to move, it wants to be stretched, so give it what it needs and, in return, it will give you what you need.

Your movement toolkit: practical, simple suggestions for daily movement

A simple yet impactful way to introduce movement is to scaffold it onto things that you're already doing on a daily basis.

* **Stretch on waking.** When we wake our natural tendency should be to rise, to stretch, to yawn, to release. If you look at any animal, or even small babies, you will see that the first thing they do when they wake is take a big yawn, roll around and stretch. We have a natural urge to move, especially after being in a fixed position while we sleep for possibly seven to nine hours. So, every morning when your feet hit the floor, take just three or four minutes to do some simple stretching. Or set your alarm 15 minutes earlier, roll out your yoga mat at the end of your bed, and do some movement or stretching.

* **Morning routines.** As you are in the bathroom brushing your teeth, you can practise some heel drops (see page 88). You could also do some gentle neck rolls, squats or hip circles.

* **Extra steps.** Park your car a bit further away from the entrance to your workplace and get those extra steps in. Perhaps you could take the stairs instead of the lift.

* **Move with others.** Make your movement a social and spiritual experience by connecting with friends or family so you are moving while also bringing joy, fun and community to the experience. Instead of meeting for a coffee this week, perhaps you and your friend could go for a walk or a run. You could also join a community-based club, such as a local tennis club or a walking group.

* **Move while waiting.** If you have children and you drop them to their sports or music class, instead of sitting in the car to wait for them, bring your runners and go for a walk or a run. Better still, get some of the other parents involved and go together! Or do some squats, burpees or monkey bar pull-ups while in the playground with your kids!

* **Dance.** My number one mood enhancer, and it's great for family bonding time. I challenge you to play some music in your bedroom or kitchen every morning and dance around like no one is watching. Let yourself just shake, bounce and be. I do this with my kids every morning and it is one of the most wonderful ways to start our day.

* **Create goals.** Set a target of 20 press-ups, sit-ups, burpees, etc. and work your way up to that, or aim to do a 5k walk or run. Having a target or goal is a super way to keep you focused and consistent.

It doesn't really matter what the movement is. As long as you are challenging yourself, committing and showing up daily, you will see your mood go up as you awaken your inner pharmacy and release those incredible chemicals in your body, boosting your self-esteem, confidence and sense of empowerment.

Over the coming weeks, can you challenge yourself to try a new form of movement? If you are used to high-intensity exercise such as running or sports, you can commit to trying something that is more breath-focused or lighter in intensity, such as yoga or Pilates. Alternatively, if you are used to doing more low-intensity exercises, you could commit to trying running, swimming or a sport that gets your heart rate up and makes you sweat.

Movement challenges and reflection

The benefits of movement are vast, for our body, mind and soul – it improves health, calms racing thoughts and brings a lightness to your soul. Over the coming month, challenge yourself to do as many of the following types of exercise as possible, or choose one from each column. Always consult your GP if you have an underlying condition or if exercise is painful. Once you have completed each of the exercises, tick the boxes to show your achievement and dedication.

High-intensity movement	Moderate- to low-intensity movement	Breath-focused movement
Running	Cycling	Yoga
Aerobics	Hiking	Pilates
HIIT circuits	Swimming	Qigong
Fast-paced dancing	Weight training/ resistance training	Nature walks/swims
Team running-based sports	Walking	Tai chi

Reflect on how each exercise made you feel.

* Was there any resistance?

* Did you find some exercises more challenging than others? If so, why?

* How can you commit to integrating different forms of movement into your weekly schedule for greater unity of mind, body and soul?

Rest, repair and recovery are the cornerstones of a balanced nervous system. Slowing down, tuning into yourself and listening your body are necessary to recharge and heal our overstimulated lives. In slowing down, we hear; in hearing, we feel; in feeling, we know. Our internal wisdom can only be heard, felt and acknowledged when we rest, repair, slow down and sleep. We must sleep in order to reap.

CHAPTER 3

OVERCOMING BROKENNESS: REST, RECOVERY, REPAIR AND SLEEP

Brokenness: when the soul screams 'Enough!'

Every one of us can relate to the feeling of being broken. Life can throw hurricanes at us – massive, life-altering catastrophes or 'big T' traumas, which inevitably leave us feeling completely broken and lost. We can also encounter many 'small T' traumas, which, when experienced consistently, can similarly make us feel fragmented, shattered, exhausted, depleted, lonely, isolated and overwhelmed.

You can feel broken if you're going through a relationship break-up – that deep devastation that unearths inner questions like, *Why me, Am I not good enough?* and *Why am I not lovable?* Or, if you're at the other end of the break-up, you might hear your inner voice asking, *Am I a bad person?* or *Am I causing guilt and pain to another person?*

We can find ourselves in this broken place due to financial pressure, if we're faced with illness, if we're grieving. I have been in this place many times and the most recent was when I became a mom: feeling exhausted, feeling you haven't a clue what you're doing, that you're wrong, incapable, useless.

In those early days of motherhood, there were some dark, deep and excruciating moments. In those first four years, sleep was rare, exhaustion was high and depletion landed at my door. There were many nights where tears fell on my tired cheeks, my eyes felt puffy, my brain was fogged, my memory was shattered, and focusing, thinking clearly or even comprehending simple things seemed impossible. Small, everyday tasks seemed mammoth and overwhelming, and I felt drained, lifeless and, ultimately, broken.

I was reading the book *The Conscious Parent* by Dr Shefali Tsabary, and somewhere between wakefulness and sleep these words came to me out of nowhere, or so it seemed, and I scribbled them down on a page in the book:

Brokenness is the ultimate exposure of one's depletion and exhaustion. It's when the spirit lacks joy or light and becomes tethered, bruised and fragmented.

When you combine relentless doing, going and 'showing' with deep-seated fatigue and disjointed or inadequate sleep, plus exposure of psychosomatic depletion, brokenness manifests. This continuous, compounding impact of overwhelm on the nervous system yields weariness, emptiness and feelings of being somewhat faulty, defeated, dispirited and, ultimately, broken.

It is always scary to expose yourself to the world, to share your vulnerabilities, for many of us are raised with the idea we should 'Put up with, show up, and wear the mask' or we shouldn't air our dirty laundry in public. We're expected to stand tall, be the best and not show our flaws. Breaking through many of my subconscious programs to share this moment so publicly is scary and raw, but it's also quite liberating. Why am I being called to share this? Because I believe there are so many other people out there who feel like this, but they have nowhere to house those feelings. I share it for all the people who feel the same, but suffer in silence for fear of shame, rejection and disapproval. For fear of being seen as stupid, weak and not capable. **If you are feeling broken, please know you are not alone. You are not weak. You are not lost. You are not even actually broken. You may feel you are, but you are simply temporarily fragmented. It is in this shattered space that the light can find a way back in, where your soul can be sewn back together and where you can be redirected back to wholeness.**

When you experience this level of fragmentation, it's almost as if God or the universe is trying to literally break you open, so that you can break down the walls of protection, the walls you were hiding behind. Maybe the life you were living wasn't serving you – whether your job, your relationship, your environment, your location, your house – and now that it's been smashed wide open, it's a great chance for change and transformation.

However, even though it presents an opportunity for growth, when you are cracked wide open you've nothing to hide behind, and all your self-worth and your inner beliefs get exposed. This is the uncomfortable point – when you want to run and hide, and revert back to the old crutches, such as over-working, over-exercising, eating too much chocolate, drinking too much wine. But if you can sit into that place and move past that sludgy, gunky part, life opens up and freedom awaits.

This place can be both the greatest and hardest opportunity of your life: the greatest because it carries such wisdom, unspoken truths and your soul's whispers; the worst because you must be honest with yourself, you must be willing to sit with all the uncomfortable, sticky emotions, and you must be willing to truly hold yourself and trust yourself in this moment. But I believe, in the long run, doing this yields greater inner confidence, courage and resilience.

It is often when you feel you have hit rock bottom that you feel a nudge, a flicker of hope that gives you the courage to turn your face towards the light and trust that you will find your way. This place of brokenness, I believe, happens for a reason: to bring you to your knees so that you have no other choice but to stop. Something in your life has been tipped too far in one direction, the scales are off balance, and your body or the universe or God is trying to give you a message, to make you listen. This makes you re-examine your entire life: your place in the world, your daily choices, your routines, your habits. You are on the stand in the trial of your own life. This can be scary, but also exciting, for if you win, you get freedom, you get to manifest your desires, you get to design a life that is true and aligned to *you*. **And you *can* win – by aligning to your truth, by listening to your heart's needs and by walking forward fearlessly through the flames that might currently appear like hell, but are, in fact, the flames that represent illumination.** It is there that your bright, glowing future awaits.

Normalise, don't stigmatise

It's important that we talk about being in this perceived broken place so that we can normalise it. Just like any time in your life when you are experiencing transition, changes or grief, the feelings can come in waves. You can be fine one moment and the next you feel like you've been struck down by a tsunami of emotion – it could be sadness, loneliness or tiredness. If we meet these emotions with love, kindness and respect, we are able to let go and create space for more 'nourishing' feelings to take their place, even just for a while.

Becoming a mom, living away from our families, moving homes and even countries several times, even though it brought so much joy to our lives, came with the stress and strain of feeling uprooted and ungrounded, which steered me in the direction of burnout.

Even though I regularly made time for my self-care – sea swims, supplements, yoga, talk therapy and movement – my experience of brokenness came from the accumulation of broken sleep, night after night, four and half years of breast-feeding, co-sleeping, giving of myself and not getting enough rest for my body and brain. The compounding impact of this on my nervous system built and built until it combusted.

Continuous pressure on the nervous system is like a bottle of fizzy water that has been shaken and shaken until the lid flies off and the water explodes everywhere. The 'water' in this case is your hormones fluctuating and your emotions being tossed around by the busyness of life. The bottle, or the vessel, is your body. This overspill of water represents a breakdown of bodily functions and the dysregulation of your nervous system.

At this time, I was meant to be writing the book you are now reading, and I had intended to have done many incred-ible things on the career front while trying to be an at-home, hands-on mother – all while moving country. **This is when my soul screamed enough** and the strain began to pull at my delicate nervous system. There came a point where I said, *No more!* I had to sit deep in my meditation practice, go into my heart and ask myself:

* What is important now?

* What do I need right now in this moment?

* What do I need to say yes to and what do I need to say no to?

* Where do my priorities lie in this moment?

* What would the best expression of my love be?

* What and where would bring me the most peace and happiness?

* What would remove stress and strain and allow me to flourish?

* What would allow me to truly listen to the whispers of my soul and the intuition of my heart?

* What lights me up?

I had to breathe and listen, cry and weep, and remove the ego that wanted me to keep going, to show the world that I could be all things to all people. I believe the greatest myth of our modern world is that women can do it all! **Perhaps we can do it all, *but at what cost?*** It could cost your relationship with your kids due to not being there for those earlier formative years, or your relationship with your partner because you are like ships in the night, or your health in the form of burnout, a dis-ease or a diagnosis.

As I sat and breathed and listened, I knew what I needed to do and where I wanted to be. My calling was to be at home with my children and to fully embrace the role of motherhood. In order to do this, I had to say no to a lot of things, but an immense relief fell over me. I could feel my lungs expand and my heart soar. I could feel spaciousness and lightness again. I felt I was coming home.

With this, of course, came difficult conversations and decisions. I had to write a letter to my editor to tell her that I could no longer write the book, that I needed to postpone it for at least a year or two. I needed to tell my husband that I was no longer going to work in our business and I needed to detach from other commitments I had agreed to at the time. Then my world opened up as I began to embrace slowing down and honouring my needs and those of my family. My life became so much more colourful, abundant and rich because I was able to truly enjoy the beauty and the bounty of being at home with my kids. As I embraced this special time, I felt nourished and oxytocin fuelled me every day, because I was honouring what my body was telling me and what my soul was yearning for. This, of course, was a decision that felt aligned to me. I know in our world today, both parents feel that they need to be working in order to survive. Sometimes we need to challenge that narrative and get creative and look at how we can rearrange life and circumstances to make it work. This of course often involves making certain changes for short phases and stages in your life, like moving house, selling a car or going part time. Making short-term changes for the long-term goal, when done with the right intention (one that feels aligned to your needs and offers nourishment to your soul), is always worth it in the long run, I believe.

Extract from the letter to Miriam's editor

I must surrender, let go of certain things in my life right now. I am in the phase of great mothering, these years I will not get back again. I cannot go on to write a book about slowing down, pausing, listening to your heart, lifestyle medicine, self-care and more if I am not 100% living and breathing the essence of the book in my own life. I must walk my talk and doing do this involves me removing myself from exhaustion and truly honouring my needs and my wellbeing.

This has been the hardest decision I have ever had to make.

It feels like a massive grief, I have cried and met places within myself that I didn't even know were there. I have never not met a deadline in my life and thus, this is what is making this so hard for me. I know however, in my heart of hearts, that this is the right decision at this present moment. Not just for me personally but for the fate of the book. If I were to write the book from this place, it wouldn't be right. It would be rushed, and possibly forced. I would be writing out of fear and lack of creativity as I am tired, and I really want the book to come from my heart and a place and space of deep reverence, meaning and an outpouring of my heart.

I feel once I come through this place, my book will be far richer, far more experiential and will have depth that I can only share once I've come through this place.

Burnout and exhaustion can't be healed over night. It takes time, permission, and a willingness to let go of certain things so that you can be put back together into wholeness.

I've also had to let go of all other work commitments for now.

The ego and my identity are screaming at me to keep pushing on, but my soul is whispering to me – not now dear one. Not now.

My soul is asking of me to Surrender, to Simplify and to Slow.

I really hope you can understand.

'When force becomes flow, the soul can say no'

Warmest love and blessings,
Miriam

How to heal from brokenness

I use the acronym BROKEN as a way to remember the key stages of how to navigate through a state of brokenness:

B – Breaks, breath, boundaries
R – Reframe, rest/repair/recovery, re-energise and revitalise, realign and redesign
O – Openness
K – Kindness
E – Engagement
N – Nourishment

The tips below really helped me in my own life, and they have helped so many clients I have worked with. I really hope they help you too.

B – breaks, breath, boundaries

Breaks

Incorporating tiny breaks into our daily life can be life-changing. Micro breaks in our day allow us to get off the treadmill, pause and come back. They give you time and space to check in and ask yourself:

* Is this the right thing for me?
* Does this feel good?
* Am I honouring my needs?
* Am I listening to my heart?

Some examples of breaks include putting your phone away for five to ten minutes, breathing for five minutes, doing a ten-minute mindfulness or meditation practice, sitting down with a warm cup of tea with no phone, book, newspaper, radio or distractions, going for a short walk in nature, taking five minutes to stretch or to journal, lighting a candle and saying a prayer.

Breath

Breathing practices have been a saving grace for me. Breathing exercises can be done anywhere, at any time. They are one of the quickest ways to rebalance your nervous system, taking you out of fight or flight and into the parasympathetic side of the nervous system (rest and repair).

Simple breathing practices that can help to realign and rebalance the nervous system and pull you out of a broken state include deep belly breathing or diaphragmatic breathing (see page 274), the 4–7–8 breath (page 275), the cooling breath (page 41), the lion's breath (page 40), the four-count box breath (page 55) or simply breathing with awareness to bring you into the present moment and take you out of the whirlwind of external chaos. The breath can make us feel grounded, unbroken and centred again, giving us courage and hope to keep going.

Boundaries

Given the complexity of human relationships, family dynamics and cultural expectations, boundaries can be one of the hardest things to set and maintain for many people (as noted in the Fawn section). It's something I must continuously work on in my own life, and it's one of the reasons I landed into such a broken state in the first place.

How are your emotional boundaries with other people? Are you a doormat? Do you let others walk all over your space and your life? Do you get bullied into making decisions that you often don't want to make but feel compelled to? Or perhaps you feel guilty if you don't comply? Do you tolerate disrespectful or hurtful behaviour? Do you speak up when someone crosses your boundaries emotionally?

Do you have healthy physical boundaries? Do you have a clear understanding around who gets into your physical space? Are your boundaries strong or are your boundaries a bit wishy-washy ?

Boundaries don't only apply to other people; we should also have boundaries with ourselves. Do you hold yourself accountable to your truth? Do you give yourself permission to stand your ground and align to your core values?

Setting healthy boundaries requires self-awareness and assertiveness. It's important that we understand our own needs and limitations, and that we communicate these limitations effectively to others in a loving and compassionate way. It may involve saying no, it may involve stepping back, speaking up and having those open and honest conversations. If we don't have clear boundaries, we risk feeling overwhelmed, resentful, burnt out, taken advantage of, emotionally drained, disconnected from ourselves and, ultimately, broken. You matter. Honesty matters. Your boundaries matter.

Practical exercise to set boundaries

Stand firmly on the ground, take a deep breath and energetically bring your awareness to your heart. Subtly and energetically imagine drawing your heart backwards, as if a magnet is gently sucking you backwards. Next imagine a ball of energy surrounding your entire body, almost like you are inside a zorb. I like to call on archangel Michael to help me create this energetic barrier. I imagine myself inside this zorb of energy and it acts as my protective shield. When someone's emotions or negative energies come towards me, I see this shield bouncing their energy back towards them, away from me, preventing me from absorbing it. Sometimes I also like to visualise a colour around them that is separate and different from mine. This creates a distance and a separation, helping me overcome 'leaky boundaries' where other energies can infiltrate my own, enabling me to feel secure and more grounded in my own energy.

R – reframe, rest/repair/recovery, re-energise and revitalise, realign and redesign

Reframe

Reframing your current situation into something more

positive helps you to look at it with fresh eyes. For example, when I was breastfeeding my children, I could easily have gone down the rabbit hole of *This is unfair, all the responsibility lies with me to bring them to bed every night, to feed them. My evenings are gone, I never get to do anything anymore.* Instead, I reframed this situation as *I get to spend this precious time bringing my kids to bed. Aren't I blessed? I get time to lie down and cuddle my babies. This is an absolute privilege. I also get to use this time to do some breathing or a lovely meditation, or have a rest and sleep.* Reframing shifts your perspective from victimhood to victory. It rephrases and repositions life in a more positive and grateful way, allowing you to see your blessings rather than engage in the complaining game, which lowers your energy levels, attracts more negative thinking in your life and ultimately gets you nowhere. When you reframe your thoughts, you move from an attitude of *I have to* to one of *I get to*. It's a completely different way of looking at life. As our tagline in Soul Space says, 'Change your thinking, change your world.'

Rest/repair/recovery

Are you giving yourself enough time to rest, recover and repair? Are you allowing yourself enough time to get out of the reactive red zone (the sympathetic side of the nervous system) and into the calm green zone (the parasympathetic side of the nervous system)?

Simple ways to rest and repair include getting adequate sleep, practising deep breathing, mindfulness or meditation, gentle exercises like yoga, walking or stretching, limiting your intake of stimulants that disrupt the nervous system, such as sugar, caffeine and alcohol, spending time in nature, listening to relaxing music, having a bath.

Re-energise and revitalise

Instead of prioritising more rest, the opposite might also be needed – perhaps when you feel broken you need more energy. Sometimes when you feel overwhelmed or depleted, you feel so exhausted and weary that you don't have the energy to do anything. Perhaps you feel you're resting all the time but still lethargic. You feel as if you have flatlined, you are in a state where you're not getting up or doing anything – perhaps you're not leaving the house, you're sleeping all the time, or you don't have the energy to get off the couch. In this state of brokenness, ask yourself, *How do I bring energy back into the body? How do I revitalise and re-energise?*

Simple ways to re-energise include drinking enough water to stay hydrated, nourishing yourself with wholefoods, reducing processed foods and stimulants, engaging in healing treatments like reflexology, acupuncture, energy work or massage, getting fresh air by opening your windows and doors, getting sunlight on your face and body, doing some cold-water therapy, even if it's as simple as splashing cold water on your face and neck, reducing negative self-talk – this can be extremely draining on the mind and body – practising positive, life-affirming affirmations, gratitude, gentle movement, stretching and deep breathing.

Realign and redesign

Taking time to realign and redesign your life is important because it allows you to reassess your goals, values and priorities. It gives you the opportunity to make necessary changes in order to create a life that lights you up.

Here are some simple ways to help you realign so you can start living from a soul-centred space:

* Reflect on what led you to brokenness. Take the time to reflect on the choices and actions that brought you to this point. Understanding the root causes of your situation can help you make more informed decisions in the future.

* Set new goals that align with your vision of what you want for your life. **We are constantly changing, renewing, evolving and maturing, so we must align our lives to match that new growth as it emerges**. Every situation teaches us something; we grow through life, so in order to not stay stuck in the past or stuck in negative patterns we must be willing to continually renew, reflect and redesign the life that we want. Take the time to regularly revisit your goals and set new ones that align with your current values and aspirations.

* Develop an action plan or create a vision board. Write it out, talk it out, draw it out. This will help you to create a clear vision or map of what will bring you more joy, inner peace and alignment. Break down your plan into smaller, manageable steps that you can take one at a time.

* Stay committed and persistent. Understand that change takes time and effort. Commit to making positive changes in your life, even when you're faced with challenges and setbacks.

Remember that being in this perceived broken place can be a turning point for growth and transformation. By taking the time to realign and redesign your life, you can create a more meaningful life for yourself.

O – openness

When you feel broken, you are cracked right open, but this 'crack' also holds the antidote. When open and broken you feel exposed, vulnerable, but it is in this exposed place that your chance awaits. When you stay open, truthful and honest, your life can transform.

This place is gifting you the chance to be your authentic self. This doesn't happen overnight; it's a process. Just as an onion has many layers, when you think you have shed every one of your layers you are met with another situation that reveals another aspect that needs healing. But the more open we are about our brokenness, the more easily we shed our layers each time and the lighter we become after each experience. When you are open you might initially recoil and think, *Oh no, why did I say that? Why did I show that side of myself? Oh my God, now they're going to hate me, or think I'm weak or weird. They're going to run a mile!* But then you will begin to realise that if they do decide to run a mile, they're not meant to be in your life. Perhaps they're not the people you need to nourish you at this time.

K – kindness

Kindness breeds compassion, self-care, self-love, and with that comes non-judgement and non-comparison. This results in us being less hard on ourselves and less critical of our actions. When we practise kindness and compassion we move through challenging times much more quickly. We ebb and flow more easily and we handle life with more grace.

Some simple ways we can be kind and compassionate to others include engaging in random acts of kindness: pay for a stranger's cup of tea in the coffee shop, send someone you love flowers or a nice card, pay someone a compliment, hold the door open for the next person, smile and say 'please' and 'thank you' to people you meet, pray and send out blessings for people who are in a difficult place. Also engage in kindness and acts of compassion for yourself by scheduling a massage or a pampering session of some sort, going for a nap, taking a rest day, unplugging, treating yourself to a warm cup of tea without distraction, having a bath, meeting up with friends, anything whereby you are honouring yourself and your needs and doing things that bring you joy and light you up.

E – engagement

Engage in things that will support you. For example, engage with your local community; take outdoor exercise; have nourishing conversations with friends, loved ones or a trained therapist; practise meditation, journalling, dancing, singing – anything that will bring a little bit of evolution, elevation and light back into your spirit. As I mentioned before, there can be a lack of light or joy in the spirit when we feel broken. **Engaging in things that help you find the light is the roadmap out of brokenness into wholesomeness.**

N – nourishment

Nourishment refers to how we can truly nourish ourselves both and off the plate. Are you feeling depleted in your life, whether nutritionally, emotionally or spiritually?

Nutritionally, are you consuming wholesome foods and beverages that are nourishing for your nervous system? Are you eating enough antioxidant-rich foods, anti-inflammatory foods, probiotic foods and magnesium to relax the body? Is your food and drink tipping your nervous system off balance, like too much caffeine, sugar, alcohol or processed foods? Are you drinking enough water? Being nutritionally fulfilled is important so that, biochemically speaking, you have the correct building blocks to make essential neurotransmitters and hormones, such as serotonin, dopamine, oxytocin and endorphins to elevate your mood and reawaken your own inner pharmacy.

What else is nourishing you or not nourishing you? Look at things beyond the plate. Is there too much stress in your life? Are you getting enough sleep? Are you having enough fun? Are you moving your body? Are you in healthy and loving relationships?

Use these practical BROKEN steps whenever you feel like you need a helping hand and a compass to help you heal from brokenness and return to wholesomeness.

Sleep: the restful recharge

Finding myself in a broken place led me to reassess the whole area of sleep and why it's such an important pillar in lifestyle medicine. Sleep is one of the body's biggest allies to health, because it allows the body to engage in its repair and restorative practices, encouraging things like cell growth and repair, and memory consolidation, as well as activating the cleansing and detoxifying processes in the body.

Sleep can be compared to a dishwasher – it is a vital process that helps to clear and refresh the mind and body. Just as a dishwasher removes grime and dirt from dishes, sleep helps to remove waste products from the brain through a process called the glymphatic system. Without proper sleep, our bodies can become overwhelmed by these waste products, leading to a decrease in cognitive function and overall health. Sleep cleanses our mind and body, enabling us to access a deeper level of our soul, allowing us to wake up feeling refreshed, rejuvenated and restored.

Sleep fits beautifully into the integrated wellbeing model, where everything is interconnected – mind, body and soul – as it has a profound impact on all three areas.

Mind

* Sleep has been shown to greatly help increase mood, concentration, focus and clarity of thought. It also reduces irritability, stress, anxiety and depression. A good quality and quantity of sleep every night enables you to awaken feeling more refreshed and more readily able to take on the day ahead.

* Sleep also has a profound impact on our memory and our ability to think clearly under pressure, as well as enabling us to make better decisions either professionally or personally.

Body

* A good quality and quantity of sleep strengthens the body's immune system. When you fall asleep, your immune system wakes up, allowing the healing and repair systems in the body to start working for you.

* Sleep decreases blood pressure and the risk of cardiovascular and heart disease.

* It can help regulate body weight and metabolism, as both of these centres are located in the same part of the brain. If you are exhausted or fatigued due to lack of sleep, your body will start to crave sugar for energy and it will do this by going for the quickest-releasing forms of glucose it can get, which is generally processed sugary foods such as buns, cakes, biscuits, scones and processed refined carbohydrates.

* Good sleep techniques can curb inflammation. Research from Emory University has shown that people who sleep

for six hours or less have higher levels of inflammatory proteins in their blood, and the root of most illnesses and disease comes from excess inflammation. Therefore, by improving and increasing your sleep, you can help reduce the risk of illness and disease.

Soul

*   If you sleep well, you wake feeling more alive, refreshed and regenerated, so you are more creative, more forward-thinking and often more enthusiastic and energetic about life, your desires and goals.

*   Rest, recovery and sleep can reignite, restore and rejuvenate a tired, weary soul.

*   A good quality and quantity of sleep allows the soul to heal and recover from the strains and stresses of daily life. It provides the soul with an opportunity to rest and recharge, promoting feelings of peace and contentment.

*   Sleep also enhances our spiritual connection. We can feel more connected to our higher selves as well as the world around us. This can lead to greater self-awareness, insight and a deeper sense of purpose.

*   During the transition from wakefulness to sleep, and again on transitioning from sleep to wakefulness, we can tap into a theta brain wave state, which is associated with deep relaxation, creativity and heightened spiritual awareness. It is often referred to as the 'God' space, because it is where individuals may experience a strong connection to their intuition, inner wisdom and higher consciousness. This theta brain wave state can serve as a sacred space for

self-discovery and healing, whereby you can tap into deeper levels of the subconscious mind, release limiting beliefs and connect to your inner guidance and spiritual essence. This is why it is very powerful to play affirmations, listen to meditations or do visualisations just as you are falling to sleep; as you enter this relaxed, hypnotic state, you can begin to reprogram your subconscious mind, plant new, positive seeds in your mind and gain deeper insight into your soul's whispers.

What is the recommended amount of sleep?

Ideally, it is recommended that adults get somewhere between seven and nine hours' sleep a night, and it has been suggested that women may, in fact, need more sleep than men, suggesting anywhere between seven and ten hours' sleep per night. Are you getting the recommended amount of sleep? If not, there could be various lifestyle factors impacting your sleep. It's important not to be hard on yourself or see it as another failure on your part. Instead, see if you can begin by developing a more loving, harmonious relationship with sleep. Here's how ...

Creating a healthy relationship with sleep

We all engage with sleep every night (hopefully), but we rarely, if ever, ask ourselves, 'What is my relationship with sleep like?' Think about your relationship with sleep and consider the following questions:

* Is it a loving one? Is it a respectful one? Is it a valued one?

* Do you commit to this relationship and treat it with reverence and love?

* Is it a non-negotiable?

* Is it a negative relationship, one where you don't value it, don't think you need it, don't trust it or give it grace? Do you neglect it?

* Do you view sleep as a form of self-care and relaxation?

* Do you dread night-time and dread sleep?

Just like any relationship, we must show up and commit to honouring it. The relationship you have with sleep is key to forming healthy habits and creating better sleep patterns, sleep quality and sleep quantity. Your beliefs about sleep can significantly impact its quality – perception is key. Believing in the importance and value of sleep can lead to a more positive attitude towards it, making it easier to prioritise and make necessary adjustments for better sleep, according to Fiona Brennan in her book *Sleep Well*. Negative beliefs or fears about sleep (such as worries about not being able to fall asleep or concerns about the consequences of poor sleep) can increase stress and anxiety levels, making it harder to relax and drift off to sleep.

In order to create a more harmonious relationship with sleep, it is important that you address any underlying issues and seek help from a healthcare professional if you are experiencing chronic sleep difficulties or suspect any underlying sleep disorders, such as insomnia or sleep apnoea. We must be willing to challenge our negative beliefs around sleep and identify any traumas we associate with it. Where did these ideas stem from? Was there a traumatic experience that unnerved your nervous system, preventing you from feeling safe enough to sleep? Safety and a balanced nervous system are key to enabling you to fall into a deep, restful sleep. It's important to seek help and support to challenge any negative beliefs like *I'm a bad sleeper*. Replacing these negative thoughts with positive affirmations will empower you to create new, consistent sleep routines and habits that can improve your sleep.

Self-compassion is also key. Please be kind to yourself as you work on this journey towards improving your sleep. Remember that creating a better relationship with sleep is a process that takes time and effort. But following the steps below and applying the tips and tricks for better sleep habits will help you greatly on the journey to achieving a more loving, harmonious relationship with sleep.

Top tips for enhanced quality and quantity of sleep

* **Room environment:** Temperature, noise levels, smell, light and comfort all make a huge difference to your sleep.

* **Temperature:** Your room should ideally be cool. If the temperature is too hot, it can affect sleep. Turn off radiators and open windows if your room is too stuffy.

* **Light:** Your room should be dark in order for melatonin, the sleep hormone, to be secreted from the pineal gland. Turn down the lights, close the curtains or invest in an eye mask.

* **Sound:** Is your bedroom too noisy? Is there loud traffic outside? Try minimising external distracting noises as much as possible. Close windows (as long as it's not too hot), listen to a guided meditation or invest in a pair of good-quality earplugs.

* **Smell:** Using aromatherapy can be an effective way of enhancing sleep. Try a few drops of essential oils like lavender, jasmine or rose on your pillow to help relax your mind and body.

* **Comfort:** Declutter your room to make sure your bedroom is a tranquil, peaceful space. Remove work or any stressful clutter from the bedroom. Replace your mattress if it is old and worn. Set yourself up for success by creating a tranquil bedroom environment.

* **The 3:2:1 rule:**
  » **Three hours before bed** ought to be your last main meal. Your body needs to rest and repair at night, and if you eat too close to bedtime, your body will need to work to digest your food.

  » **Two hours before bed** remove yourself from anything too taxing on the body, such as high-intensity exercise, work emails, or anything stressful. The two hours before bed is a time for winding the system down, not revving it up.

  » **One hour before bed** remove technology from your bedroom. It is said that the blue light from these devices can affect the secretion of melatonin (which is only released when it gets dark), so these bright lights can affect your ability to sleep properly. That's not to mention the destructive impact of doom-scrolling before bed can have on your mental health.

* **Create a nightly routine and establish an adult curfew:** Treat your sleep routine as you would a child's by trying to go to bed at the same time every night. This may require a period of retraining yourself. Like any sport or hobby, in

order to become good at it, you have to practise. You must be patient and persistent and have an underlying need to want to create a better night-time routine.

* **Hormonal-, emotional- or stress-related issues:** An inability to get to sleep or to stay asleep could have underlying emotional, hormonal or perimenopausal issues that needs to be addressed. If there are too many stress hormones flooding the system, it can affect our ability to sleep. Therefore, addressing your stress is vital. Trying things like meditation, deep breathing, yoga, getting out in nature, talk therapy, reducing stimulants (caffeine, alcohol, sugars, processed foods), as well as addressing any dis-harmonious issues that may be playing on your mind from a lifestyle perspective (work, relationships, etc.), will benefit your sleep.

* **Electromagnetic fields (EMFs):** These are produced by various electronic devices such as mobile phones, Wi-Fi routers and power lines. EMFs can potentially affect sleep by disrupting the body's natural circadian rhythm and interfering with the production of melatonin. Be conscious of the mobile devices and other technology that may be turned on in your bedroom. Do you sleep with your phone turned on or charging beside your bed? Ideally, your phone should be left outside your bedroom. If you need it in the bedroom, try keeping it away from the bed and having it switched to flight mode. Consider unplugging your Wi-Fi modem at night too.

* **Stimulants and supplements:** For better-quality sleep, it is advisable to reduce your stimulants, in particular caffeine, from noon onwards. Try substituting tea or

coffee with hot water and lemon or a relaxing herbal tea like chamomile.

* **Cleansing techniques and night-time rituals:** A hot epsom salts bath or a shower before bed can act as a purifying or cleansing routine to wash away the day. It can work for some people as a way to clear away unwanted conversations, thoughts or worries they might have had that day.

* **Journalling** and gratitude are other great ways of cleansing or clearing out any unwanted thoughts or stuck emotions from the mind. There's more about these in the Mind section. The energy you go to bed with is often said to be the energy you wake up with.

* **Prayer, deep breathing and meditation** are also powerful night-time rituals to incorporate into your routines for enhanced sleep quality and quantity.

Establishing a healthy sleep routine is an extremely important thing to do for your health and wellbeing.

Find a routine that suits you and your lifestyle. Remember, you don't just arrive at sleep; you must prepare for it by winding down your mind and body by practising some of these night-time routines and rituals.

Prioritising rest, sleep and repair are not just luxuries we can indulge in when we have the time: they are vital components of a healthy lifestyle that we must unapologetically prioritise. Giving ourselves the opportunity to recharge and rejuvenate makes us better equipped to face the challenges of each day with clarity, energy and reverence. Your day starts the night before, so let's make a conscious effort to value and make time for these important aspects of self-care, recognising the profound impact they have on our wellbeing and our quality of life.

True nourishment involves the integration of mind, body and soul to fuel sustainable vitality and wellbeing. Nourishment for the body focuses on the foods we eat. Nourishment for the mind focuses on the thoughts we think. Nourishment for the soul focuses on the love, joy and passion in our lives. True nourishment transcends what's on the plate. It goes far beyond the foods we eat or the nutrients we ingest.

CHAPTER 4

NUTRITIONAL WELLBEING AND OUR RELATIONSHIP WITH FOOD

This chapter is not what you might expect. It will not contain recipes or lists of ingredients – you can easily access that information in many other books and online. It will take more of a deep dive into the background behind nutrition, both on and off the plate, and, more importantly, into your relationship with the food you eat every day. We will explore nutrition not just from a physical point of view, but transcend that to show you how important nutrition is from an emotional, mental, psychological and spiritual perspective.

We will explore the concepts of what we eat, why we eat, when we eat and where we eat. We will look at food beyond the plate, exploring **soul food** and **the dance between health and happiness.** We will also journey through the fascinating world of emotional eating and eating in unwanted ways, lifting the lid and searching more deeply into how everything is connected – and how our food choices, habits and behaviours can be directly linked to the quality of our mental, physical and spiritual health. We will also explore the importance of our gut health and hydration, and I will share some simple yet powerful tips and principles for 'life and soul nourishment' to help you regain a better, more harmonious relationship with yourself and with food.

This chapter is also a very personal one for me, as I will share my own journey towards healing a fractured relationship with food. I really hope that it will help others along their journey to healing their relationship with themselves and with their plate.

The transformational power of food: the holy grail

In a world filled with endless distractions and temptations, it can be easy to overlook the profound impact that our food choices have on our overall wellbeing. The ancient wisdom of Hippocrates still rings true today: 'Let food be thy medicine and medicine be thy food.' To add to this, Dr Mark Hyman says, 'Let thy kitchen be thy pharmacy,' which, as a pharmacist, I absolutely love.

As we navigate through the busy demands of our lives, it is essential to remember that one of the keys to health and vitality lies in the food we consume.

I always had a deep-seated awareness, even from an early age, that what we put into our body has to impact how it works, reacts and responds. If you have a car and you don't take care of it, it will break down. If you put the wrong fuel or dirty fuel into the car, it will not function properly and begin to break down. The same is true of our bodies. Our bodies are sacred temples that need food not just to fuel us but also to allow us to thrive so we can feel amazing, have life-force energy and be free from many modern-day diseases.

For many of us, myself included, cultivating a healthy relationship with food is a journey of self-discovery and healing. In a society that relies on ultra-processed and chemical-laden foods, it can be challenging to prioritise nourishing our bodies and souls with wholesome, real foods. However, as I have learned through my own experiences, **making the conscious choice to eat more mindfully and healthily is not only a necessity, but a sacred act of self-care and self-love**.

Unfortunately, convenience culture and powerful marketing often trumps nutrition, making it easy to fall into the trap of relying on pre-packaged and processed foods. However, we must remember that our bodies are our temples, and they deserve the highest-quality fuel. By choosing to nourish ourselves with wholesome, natural and nutrient-dense foods, we not only support our physical health, but also nurture our emotional and spiritual wellbeing.

Food today, unfortunately, is not the same as it was years ago. We often hear our parents or grandparents saying, 'Oh sure, I ate that growing up' or 'We used to give that to you guys as kids all the time and aren't you all okay?' Yes, that may ring (slightly) true, but many of the foods and the ingredients in food products today are dramatically different from how they used to be. They have changed significantly over the past few decades – in how they are grown, farmed, prepared and produced.

There are several factors that have changed how food is produced. There's been an industrialisation of agriculture, which has led to a shift towards large-scale industrial farming methods. This has led to widespread use of pesticides, herbicides and synthetic fertilisers, which can have negative impacts on both our environment and our health. The food industry has also become increasingly reliant on processed and packaged foods, which are often high in sugar (and artificial sugars), salt and unhealthy fats. These foods may be convenient and affordable, but they are costly to our health in the long term, as they lack essential nutrients and contribute to the rise of diet-related issues such as obesity, diabetes and heart disease. These changes have resulted in a food chain system that prioritises convenience, efficiency and profit over nutrition, health and sustainability.

Overfed and undernourished

In a world of abundance and excess, it is paradoxical that so many of us are suffering from a lack of true nourishment. We find ourselves caught in a vicious cycle of overconsumption, yet our bodies (and souls) are starved of the essential nutrients needed to thrive. This phenomenon, known as being overfed and undernourished, is an epidemic that plagues our society.

We are eating 'food-like products' that are high in calories, sugar, chemicals, artificial ingredients and predominantly made in a lab, but these foods are devoid of any real nutrients, vitamins and minerals. So, even though we are eating lots of food, deep down, our cells are not getting everything they need to grow, repair and thrive. This can lead to cravings and the body being constantly hungry. You end up eating more and more food-like products, but your body is actually depleted and undernourished.

Being overfed and undernourished is not only a physical ailment but also a lifestyle and spiritual crisis. Beyond the plate, we can be overfed with things in our life that are damaging to our health. For example, we can be overfed long hours of work and we can be undernourished in rest and recovery. We can be overfed stress and strain and be undernourished in joy, laughter, play and fulfilment. We can be overfed negative self-talk, judgement, criticism, blame and shame and we can be undernourished in compassion, forgiveness and love.

When we continually deprive ourselves of essential nutrients, our bodies begin to cry out for real, whole foods that nourish us at a cellular level. But often these cries are suppressed or ignored because the build-up of toxicity from ultra-processed foods blocks the gut from sending us those intuitive messages. It is only when we quieten down the mind and nourish ourselves with wholesome real foods that we get to hear these calls of wisdom from our cells and our soul.

As a holistic health practitioner, I have witnessed the detrimental effects of the overfed and undernourished phenomenon. The symptoms of this imbalance manifest in various forms, including fatigue, mood swings, digestive issues and chronic disease. However, I firmly believe that one of the key 'ingredients' to true healing is a return to the roots of conscious eating and a deep reverence for the power of real food.

As we journey through this chapter, we will learn how to break free from the cycle of being overfed and undernourished to embrace a life of greater simplicity, consistency and fulfilment.

The sacred dance of food and health: nourishing our bodies, minds and souls

We must remember that **we are nature**. We are not robots planted here in the natural world; we are part of the natural world. When we eat food that is not natural, our bodies (which are natural beings) find it extremely difficult to understand, connect and digest these artificial ingredients and products. This disconnect wreaks havoc on our digestive system, immune function and overall wellbeing. The consequences of such dietary choices can be far-reaching, and lead to chronic inflammation, hormonal imbalances and a host of preventable diseases.

The impact of food on our health extends beyond the physical realm; it also influences our mental and emotional wellbeing. A diet rich in whole, plant-based foods is known to support mental clarity, emotional resilience and overall cognitive function, as we will see when we explore the gut–brain axis (see page 169). By nourishing our brains with essential nutrients and antioxidants, we can enhance our focus, memory and mood, fostering a state of vibrant mental health.

It is crucial to recognise that our bodies are not only physical vessels but also spiritual temples, requiring real and harmonious nourishment to thrive. As we awaken to the truth that food is not merely sustenance but a potent form of healing, we empower ourselves to reclaim our inner pharmacy.

By cultivating a deep reverence for the power of real, whole foods, we can unlock the transformative potential of food as medicine. Each bite becomes a prayer, each meal becomes a sacred communion, an act of self-love that reverberates through us on every level: body, mind, and soul.

The four Ws

When it comes to integrative nutrition, which involves a holistic approach to nourishing ourselves back to wholeness, it is important to look beyond just what we eat. We need to take a broad-spectrum approach:

* **Where** we eat
* **When** we eat

* **What** we eat
* **Why** we eat.

Where are we eating?

We consume far more than the food on our plates; we also digest and consume the environment in which we are eating. Do you eat in a stressful environment? In a noisy place? At your desk? In the car? On the go? Maybe you eat while watching TV or reading the news or scrolling through your phone. If so, you are likely to be distracted, which makes you more likely to eat without awareness and overeat. If you eat in a stressful environment (for example at your desk) your digestion will be disrupted. This is because, as we learned in the Stress chapter, when you are in a state of stress, your body is more concerned with keeping you safe than digesting your food, so your digestive function gets down-regulated.

Tips to improve the 'where'

* Eat mindfully. Pause, breathe and be grateful for the food you are about to eat.

* Practise grace and gratitude. Pause before you eat, say grace, give thanks for the food you are about to eat. Be mindful of where it has come from, the hands that have made it and prepared it. Become conscious of how lucky you are to have this abundant, beautiful food to nourish your cells. Send love and thanks to your digestive organs for all the incredible work they do for you every day to keep you healthy and alive.

* Chew your food. Remember, you have no teeth past your mouth!

* Don't eat at your desk or on the go. Slow down and take time for your meals. Enjoy your food and make mealtime a ritual.

* Engage in nourishing conversations at mealtimes. Avoid confrontation or arguments while eating. Remember, you ingest and digest the environment and energy in which you are eating.

* Unplug from phones and make mealtimes at home and at work a tech-free space.

When are we eating?

The timing of our meals is just as important as the quality of the food we eat. Establishing a consistent eating pattern that works for you, such as consuming three balanced meals a day with healthy snacks in between, can have numerous benefits for overall wellbeing – but we are all different, so finding a pattern that works well for you is key.

Do you eat regularly throughout the day? Or do you leave long gaps between meals? This can lead to adrenaline becoming your go-to source of energy or fuel instead of glucose – and adrenaline is one of your stress hormones. So, in effect, you may be fuelling yourself with adrenaline rather than nutrition. If we are living off adrenaline, this can lead to extra pressure and stress being placed on our adrenal glands, thus overstimulating our nervous system. In the long term this can have a destructive impact on our health, physically, mentally and emotionally.

A benefit of establishing a regular eating routine is maintaining stable blood sugar levels throughout the day. By spacing meals and snacks evenly and not skipping meals, we can prevent energy crashes, mood swings and cravings for unhealthy foods. This can also help regulate our metabolism and promote healthy weight management.

Another key aspect of meal timing is avoiding eating too late at night. Consuming heavy meals close to bedtime can disrupt our natural sleep cycle and digestion process, leading to poor-quality sleep and weight gain.

Think about how you start your day. The word 'breakfast' means 'breaking the fast'. This is why people often refer to breakfast as one of the most important meals of the day. What do you allow into your body to break this fast, and when?

Seasonal eating can be a great way of bringing together the 'what' and the 'when' of eating together. Try to buy locally and eat with the seasons, which aligns the body with the natural rhythms of nature and helps to maintain optimal balance and health. For example, consuming warm, soothing foods like soups and stews in winter, but eating cooler salads and juices in the summer months, is conducive to greater digestion.

Seasonal foods are naturally more nourishing as they are at their peak of freshness and contain more nutrients. As the seasons change, so do our bodies, so eating in tune with the seasons can help us flow more easily and adapt to these changes.

Tips to improve the 'when'

*   Find an eating pattern that specifically *works for you*, one that keeps you sustained and energised throughout the day.

*   Avoid long gaps between meals (unless you are fasting) to reduce overeating and cravings.

* Try something like hot water and lemon in the morning to help cleanse and detoxify the body. Avoid breaking your fast with stimulants like caffeine or sugar, as this will disrupt your blood sugar levels.

* Have your last meal at least two to three hours before bedtime. Reduce or cut out caffeine and sugars in the afternoon and evening to improve sleep and energy levels.

* Buy locally and eat with the seasons.

What are we eating?

Bio-individuality

Bio-individuality means that we are all different – no one diet is universally right; there are no hard-and-fast rules that work for everyone. Experiment and see what works best for you.

I use a concept called JERF, or Just Eat Real Food. It sounds so simple and may seem like common sense, but unfortunately this concept isn't that common in our world of 'grab and go' convenience food. JERF means going back to basics: back to eating food that is real, food that comes from the ground or grows on trees, and fewer processed or chemically modified foods.

* Eat more food that is colourful and alive. Healthy, vibrant, living foods are filled with energy, so they give you energy.

* Reduce ultra-processed foods that come in packages and plastic. If the food is dead, or processed, there is no life there; it is not likely to bring a renewed sense of life to you or your cells.

* Reduce caffeine, sugars and processed foods and include more of Mother Earth's plants (fruits and vegetables, nuts, seeds, herbs, spices) to obtain a wholesome and nutritious diet.

Crowding out

I learned this concept when I was studying with the Institute for Integrative Nutrition and it opened my eyes to how we can really nourish ourselves, rather than just trying to feed ourselves.

There is a big difference between nourishment and simply fuelling the body. When we nourish ourselves, it evokes a feeling of wanting to take care of ourselves. To me, the word 'nourishment' means deep reverence, it means deep care, and it highlights a loving relationship with food. To me, simply fuelling or feeding the body signifies a duty rather than a passion. You're fuelling your body so that you can perform or succeed, so that you can be active and have energy, but nourishment has more of a soulful reverence – a feeling of being nurtured with love and care.

The concept of 'crowding out' eliminates a 'lack and limitation' mindset, or a diet mindset. When you're living with a diet mindset, you're constantly trying to cut everything out, reduce, remove: *Don't eat that!* It breeds starvation and deprivation. This does not say nourishment to me. It screams despair and disconnection. Crowding out, however, means that you keep 'adding in' – adding in more of the beneficial stuff. For example, add in more green leafy vegetables, fruit, water, nuts, seeds, spices, root vegetables ... If you keep adding and adding and adding nourishment to your plate, it will eventually crowd out the stuff that's serving you less – sugars, processed food, trans fats, etc. As you eat more wholesome foods, your tastebuds will change. You will crave more of the healthy, nutritious, wholesome foods and you will feel fewer cravings for sugar and processed foods.

The concept of 'crowding out' can also go beyond the plate. You can add in more things like exercise and movement, and crowd out sitting on the couch, scrolling on your phone or watching mindless TV. You can add in more meditation and breathwork and crowd out stress and worry. You can add in more rest and repair and crowd out busyness and rushing. You can add in more dance, play, community and fun and crowd out sadness, loneliness and depression. Crowding out will result in a life that's filled with true nourishment, fulfilment and joy.

The rainbow plate

Ideally, the food on your plate ought to be full of colour, resembling a rainbow (greens, yellows, reds, purples, orange, etc.) and be predominately plant-based (fruits and vegetables). These colourful foods are packed with phytochemicals, vitamins, minerals and fibre that support immune function and gut health, promote heart health and reduce inflammation.

Incorporating the rainbow diet into your life will allow for greater health, energy and vitality.

Read the labels

One of the most important things you can do for your nutritional wellbeing is to learn how to read the labels on your food. Reading labels is crucial when making good food choices as, unfortunately, marketing tactics can often be misleading. Many food products on the market are packed and advertised in a way that make them appear healthier than they are, when they might actually be loaded with hidden sugars, unhealthy fats or artificial additives. Terms like 'natural' or 'low fat' can be misleading when they are not backed up by the actual ingredients on the label. By taking the time to understand food labels, you can make educated choices about the products you consume.

Pay attention to the nutritional facts, read the ingredients list and check serving sizes to ensure that you are making the best choices for you and your family. It only takes a few seconds to turn the product around and read the ingredients. These seconds may make a huge difference to your health in the long term.

How to read food labels

*   Never believe the front cover! Just because it has the word 'nature' or 'natural' in it doesn't mean it is healthy.

*   Follow the 'rule of five'. Products should ideally contain five ingredients or fewer. If a label has a long list of ingredients, many of which are chemical and artificial, it is a clear indicator that the product isn't healthy or natural.

*   If you can't pronounce it, you probably shouldn't be eating it!

*   Pay attention to the order of the list: the first ingredient on the list is present in the largest amount. If sugar is the first ingredient listed, the product is mainly made of sugar.

*   Be aware of artificial sweeteners, which are often listed under 'Carbohydrates (of which sugars)' on the label. They may remove the sugar content from the product but will replace it with chemicalised sweeteners instead, such as aspartame, glucose syrup, high fructose corn

syrup, sucrose, dextrose, fructose, maltose or malto-dextrin. Many of these are not natural and are often made in a lab, which wreaks havoc on our digestive system and immune system. These are often found in 'diet' drinks and products.

* Be aware of diet and fat-free products. In these products the fat is removed but it is often replaced by fake or chemicalised sweeteners and salt. They are not a healthier option.

* Know how to read the sugar content on labels. The recommended daily amount of sugar is six teaspoons for women and eight for men. A teaspoon of sugar is about 4g. For example, a can of Coke contains 39g of sugar, which is the equivalent of nine teaspoons of sugar per can! So just one sugary soft drink can put you over the recommended daily limit.

* Watch out for serving sizes. Many packaged foods contain multiple servings, so be sure to evaluate the serving size listed on the label to accurately gauge the nutritional content that you are consuming.

Having said that, be careful not to become obsessive, which can lead to more stress on the body. Having the awareness to make healthy and informed decisions is key, but so too is balance. Sometimes having that bar of chocolate or that glass of wine is okay, and it might be less stressful than constantly having to get everything right or always make your diet perfect!

Why are we eating? The void within

We all know at some level what we think we should be eating: less sugar and cake and more fruits and vegetables. But if we already know this, *why* don't we do it? I believe this comes down to our relationship with food, our relationship with ourselves and the concept of emotional eating. We might feel compelled to eat more than we need or food that we know isn't good for us, or we might restrict our intake of food altogether. This can come in the form of overeating and yo-yo dieting, or our relationship with food might progress to dysregulated binge eating or anorexia. Whether you overeat or under-eat isn't really the issue; **what's driving the disharmonious relationship with food is an underlying emotional disruption**. Often a wounded inner child who is looking for protection, safety, love and acceptance. A belief system that has been bruised and possibly broken, either through years of everyday small-T traumas or a large-T trauma that led to a wounded self-image where you don't feel like you're good enough. This creates an inner void, a hole in the soul, which we try to fill with external substances (often food) in an attempt to build us up again, to make us feel unbroken and to make us feel 'hole-some' again. Emotional eating is a complex subject, and one I have personal experience in, so let's graciously explore this area around our relationship to food.

Primary versus secondary foods

Learning about the concept of primary and secondary foods at the Institute for Integrative Nutrition was truly awe-inspiring. It enabled me to re-evaluate my relationship with food. It brought me greater inner ease, and allowed my body weight to gravitate back to my natural size without strain, struggle or effort. Once I cleaned up my inside world and fuelled myself with *soul* foods, everything came back into alignment.

Primary food: soul food

When I ask 'What are primary foods?' during my keynote talks, a lot of hands go up and people usually respond that a primary food is one from a core nutrient group, for example a carbohydrate or a healthy fat, or water. However, primary foods are not food at all.

Primary foods cannot be found on a plate. They are all the things that truly nourish you, that energise you, that make you feel fulfilled, that are not found in meals. When we talk about food, we typically think of the food we eat. But the integrated approach also considers other 'food' that sustains our life: the things that give us joy, meaning or fulfilment and make life worth living. These foods are called primary or soul foods.

Finding primary foods involves looking outside the realm of food, beyond the plate, for nourishment. Remember, food is not the issue; food is the symptom. The issue is often caused by the void within. Finding primary food involves looking beyond the external to your internal world. What is your soul seeking? Which 'food' would nourish your soul? What are you hungry for? We often hunger for things like more play, fun, adventure, freedom, courage, confidence, achievement, success, love, intimacy, touch, art, music, rest, community, self-expression, leadership, excitement or spirituality. All these elements are essential forms of nourishment, none of which you can pick off a shelf and put onto your plate. The extent to which we are able to incorporate these soul foods into our lives determines how worthwhile and joyful we feel.

Think about a child playing outside with their friends, laughing, joking, jumping, running – they are truly exhilarated. When their mother calls them in for dinner, they don't hear her, because at that moment, what's really nourishing the child, what's really bringing their soul alive, is the connection, the fun, the laughter, the sense of adventure. All of these incredible things will never be found on a plate. These are true primary or soul foods.

Primary foods can also come in the form of a hug from a loved one when you are feeling anxious, or the calm you feel after a long talk with a friend. It's the smell of freshly baked bread in your nana's house, getting a promotion at work or seeing your child walk for the first time. It's that swim in the sea, that warm soak in the bath or curling up with a good book. It is said that sometimes we are not fed by the food on our plate but by the energy in our lives.

These primary soul foods can be categorised into **four main pillars**.

1. Relationships

What's your relationship with yourself like? When you look in the mirror, what do you tell yourself? How do you speak to yourself every day? The more negative or harsh we are with ourselves, the more we create internal toxicity that leads to outbursts of self-sabotage and self-punishment, overeating being a typical repercussion of this.

What's your relationship with others like? Do you carry grudges or have enemies? Are there lingering issues in particular relationships that form disharmonious feelings, and can these be repaired? Do you need to forgive someone or ask for forgiveness? Harbouring guilt, shame, anger or blame creates disharmony in the mind and body. It results in an inner world of conflict. This fractured energy breeds unhappiness and, as a result, often fuels destructive behaviours.

Who do you surround yourself with? Do you surround yourself with people that inspire you and encourage you to grow? Or do you hang around with people who dim your light, don't appreciate you and your accomplishments, or who are toxic for your soul?

2. Career

Are you in a job that you are truly passionate about and that lights you up? Do you love what you do? Does it energise you? Does it bring a smile to your face? Is what you're doing of service to people? If the answer to any of these questions is no, ask yourself what you need to do to bring more life to this pillar of primary food. You don't necessarily have to take drastic measures like changing your career or quitting your job (though sometimes people do!); there are other smaller things you can do, such as moving department, finding a different position in your company or even something as simple as decluttering your desk.

Ask yourself what brought you to this career in the first place. Can you rekindle that spark? What has extinguished your passion? Maybe you are just tired or in need of a fresh start. Or maybe your soul is screaming at you to do something else, follow your dreams, pursue a passion. If so, what small steps can you put in place to flow in the direction of your heart's desire?

When we are not aligned in our career or in our purpose, we feel internal disharmony. The more disharmony we feel internally, the more the void within grows and we therefore turn to things to soothe ourselves, such as food.

3. Physical activity

Do you have regular movement in your life? It is essential that we move the body, not just for weight management or to achieve a particular physique, but also to move out emotions and to elevate our mood and mental wellbeing (as discussed in Chapter 2). Remember, the word emotion (e-motion) means energy in motion. Our emotions are meant to be moved out of the body.

4. Spirituality and heeding the call of your soul

Your soul is your inner spark of light. It is your essence. It's your characteristics. It's your dreams, your passions, your desires. True health and happiness stem from living a life that is aligned with your soul's script and to your inner callings.

Embracing spiritual wellbeing means different things to different people. It might be getting out in nature, having a bath, going for a swim in the ocean, rolling out your yoga mat, meeting up with friends and having a good laugh, or connecting to God or the universe through prayer, silence and meditation.

We will explore spiritual health in greater detail in the Soul section of the book.

Secondary food

The food we eat is what we call secondary food, and of course it's very important. We want to eat healthy, natural, wholesome foods as much as possible. Essentially, we need to fill up on both sources (primary and secondary) to feel truly well. Whenever we aren't feeling healthy or something feels 'off', it could be the result of an imbalance of either our primary or our secondary foods. We all know that if something's not going well in our relationship or career, it can lead to changes in mood, which can often drive cravings and unhealthy eating patterns, leading to a whole host of health issues such as digestive problems, weight gain, diabetes, etc.

So, while it's important to eat local, varied, organic food, having balance in the other areas of your life and a good dose of passion for things that feed your mind, inspire

your heart and awaken your soul is just as important for maintaining good health. As I learned in the Institute for Integrative Nutrition, 'When primary food is balanced and satiated, your life feeds you, making what you eat secondary.'

Balancing the primary foods

I like to think of the four pillars of your primary foods (relationships, physical activity, career, spirituality) as like the four tyres on your car. If one of your tyres gets a puncture, but you ignore it, continue driving and say to yourself, *It's okay, there is a great petrol station up ahead and it has the best petrol in the world, there are no toxins or pollutants in it, it's completely clean fuel. I'll fill up my tank there, and I won't bother fixing the tyre – that will get me to my destination on time*, you won't get too far down the road. Your primary foods are your foundation in life, like the tyres on your car. If they're not filled with air, if your soul is not filled with love, your life will seem flat and weary. Just as tyres can get flat and worn out, we too can get flat and worn out. We need to constantly refill the 'air' in our lives, our primary foods, so that we can be at our best and create inner harmony, coherence and ease.

We can be putting the best fuel into the car by eating the best food in the world (secondary food), but if we are out of balance in one or two or even all four of our primary food pillars, we won't be fully healthy or fully happy.

For me, realising this was a lightbulb moment. At the height of my emotional eating, two of my primary pillars were askew, causing a conspicuous imbalance in my life. It felt as though I was driving aimlessly, the two flat tyres hindering my ability to navigate smoothly towards success, fulfilment, peace and joy. It is no surprise that during that period my overall wellbeing and performance were not at their peak.

I started to clean up my internal world, rebalance my pillars, find my passion again and make some big decisions around career and relationships. And then, almost like magic, the compulsion to seek solace in external sources of nourishment waned; the need to stuff myself with secondary food dissipated. I started to become free from the caged world of emotional eating and reclaimed a newfound sense of liberation.

Emotional eating

The most toxic of all food is toxic thoughts. The greatest digestive issues arise not just from the food on our plate but from undigested emotions and unreleased trauma.

If you are reading this and have had your struggles with food, with body image, with weight, or you know a loved one who has struggled or is still struggling with any of these areas, know that I hear you, I see you, I feel your pain. I know this path only too well, as I have walked it myself and lived through it with others. I know how destructive it can be – not just physically, but mentally. It can feel like you're living in a pressure cooker, where food becomes your biggest enemy yet also your greatest source of comfort.

So what is emotional eating? How does it show up? Why do we do it? And how can we break the cycle and overcome it in a healthy way?

My personal story weaves beautifully into what I do now in my professional life, which is help people move out of a conflicting relationship with food, allowing them to recreate love of self, reignite their image of brilliance, be free of restrictions, rigidity and fears, and, above all, develop a relationship with food that is healthy, loving, respectful and harmonious.

My journey began in my late teens and early 20s when I was in college, and my whole world focused on the external. I was studying pharmacy, which focuses solely on the physical body. It looks at health and wellbeing from a mechanical, Newtonian physics point of view, where everything is seen as matter, often disregarding or ignoring the potency of energy and emotions for our physical wellbeing.

All the while, I was trying to find myself in the world. I began sourcing my sense of value, purpose and meaning from how I appeared to the world on the outside. I became consumed by my physicality. My priority, worth and importance became solely focused on how I looked, how much I weighed, my body shape, what size clothes I wore, how many calories I consumed and how many calories I burnt off on the treadmill. I became a slave to the world of yo-yo dieting. The horrendous roller-coaster of ups and downs, being flung from pillar to post, mentally, emotionally and physically, and becoming a prisoner of the rigid rules I had created for myself. These rules reinforced my own pain, punishment and self-defeat, because deep down I perceived that I was unworthy, incapable and somewhat useless. Anything over a size 8 was seen as a failure in my eyes; being skinny was my prize, my Olympic medal. If I was the thinnest, the prettiest, the most glamorous, then surely I'd be seen, liked, approved of and would consequently feel successful, happy and, dare I say, 'worthy'. This dangerous path I walked led to years of horrendous self-talk, self-sabotage, escapism, denial, frustration and perfectionism.

In the lead-up to my pharmacy finals, I found myself in a very anxious state. My nervous system was extremely heightened, and I was in a state of fear that almost paralysed me.

I couldn't eat, I couldn't sleep, I was a nervous wreck. I was studying around the clock. Even though I loved what I was learning, I hated it too, for it was making me sick – because deep down I feared failure and what might happen if I didn't succeed or pass my exams. There was a voice inside my head shouting loudly, tossing me into the sympathetic side of the nervous system that made me a prisoner of fear. This fear caused anxiety, which led to appetite suppression, sleep disturbances, constant butterfly feelings in my tummy and a relentless need to exercise to escape from these nervous feelings.

Once the exams were finished, what happened? The big release: my shoulders dropped, the butterflies vanished and, as my friends would say, 'bungee Miriam' appeared! Like someone doing a bungee jump, I was carefree and fun. I was just finding a way to vent, to release the fear, to escape.

While this felt amazing at the time, a recoil effect often followed. This recoil effect is like drinking too much alcohol – you're likely to feel dreadful the next day. Similarly, if you eat too much, you experience feelings of shame, guilt, disgust and even disgrace. Have you ever experienced a 'food coma' after Christmas dinner? After you have eaten too much food, you slump on the couch, feeling exhausted, swollen, tired and flat. Even though you might feel overfull, the likelihood is that you will end up going back for more food (maybe some turkey sandwiches or mince pies) a few hours later, and the cycle repeats.

Your stomach, of course, is a muscle as well as an organ, so as you eat more, the muscle expands and creates more space, causing you to feel hungry all the time. However, this is just a physical side effect or by-product of overeating. The root cause is where the real healing is found. This Christmas Day experience might be a once-off for some people, but for anyone struggling with their relationship to food and subsequently with their weight, it can be an everyday occurrence. It's exhausting and painful and debilitating on every level – physically, mentally, emotionally and spiritually. This suppression breeds depression and often yields a split from the soul – from the heart of who you are.

For me, each release was met with a recoil effect. A self-directed shaming, berating and shunning that left a scar. This wound was filled with feelings of not being enough and of humiliation.

The reason I'm sharing this story about my final exams is to share what happened next: I found myself in a very scary position; I became critically unwell.

After my finals, I headed off with a group of girls, backpacks in tow, to travel in Southeast Asia for the summer. After navigating the demands of the final exams, the prospect of travelling seemed like a much-needed escape. However, amidst the adrenaline of travelling and experiencing unforgettable adventures, I found myself neglecting my basic needs, particularly when it came to nourishing my body. Battling the pressures of exams had already taken a toll on my physical wellbeing, leaving me severely underweight. Despite being aware of my fragile body, the distraction of exploration combined with my disharmonious relationship with food led me to overlook the importance of proper nutrition, because to me feeling thin was the greatest meal of all. In the depths of my struggle with undernourishment, the elusive pursuit of thinness overshadowed the basic human need for sustenance, offering a false sense of satisfaction and control. As I got thinner and my health deteriorated, the emptiness became a twisted substitute for nourishment, a toxic cycle of self-deprivation and self-deception. **It was only through the harsh reality of the severity of my illness that I came to**

understand the value of health and vitality, realising that true fulfilment lies not in the emptiness of thinness, but in the richness of a life well-lived.

As the weight continued to drop off, my body began to show visible signs of distress. My already compromised immune system succumbed to the unforgiving grip of bilateral pneumonia, a harsh consequence of my negligence.

On returning home, I was extremely unwell and breathless, and at the tender age of 21 I ended up in ICU, battling for each laboured breath. Now I was faced with the stark reality of my fragility. The once vibrant and adventurous spirit that drove me to embark on the journey had become frail and vulnerable. Surrounded by beeping machines and concerned medical professionals, I found myself grappling with the repercussions of my own actions. The warmth of Southeast Asian sunsets was replaced by the sterile walls of a hospital room.

It was in those dark moments that I came to understand the gravity of my choices. The reckless abandonment of my own wellbeing in pursuit of fleeting pleasures had brought me to this horrific place, a sobering realisation that left me reeling. As I fought to regain my strength and rebuild my fragile body, I vowed to never again take my health for granted. The harrowing experience taught me the invaluable lesson of self-care. It gave me a new appreciation for the gift of health and the resilience of the human spirit.

Fast forward a year. I had recovered from my pneumonia and regained my strength and my health physically, but I had not healed emotionally or psychologically. Thus my relationship with food took a whole new route. Instead of eating in unwanted ways (under-eating) as I had previously, the pendulum began to swing in the opposite direction, and I began to overeat or binge. I began practising as a pharmacist and this is when it became obvious that my disharmonious relationship with food was once again out of control. This obsessive way of living continued as I travelled to Australia, New Zealand and Bali – no matter where in the world I went, my inner world came with me. You can never outrun what's inside you. You have to meet it head-on with compassion, curiosity, understanding, forgiveness and grace.

One day, sitting on the floor in my sister's house, not long after returning home from Australia, I let the mask fall. I no longer denied my disharmonised internal state. I wept uncontrollably, realising there and then that I needed help. I surrendered to the fact that this wasn't normal and that I could no longer go on living like this.

This journey brought me to my greatest healer, friend, support: Brighid. Brighid is an exceptional biodynamic psychotherapist who took me under her wing and stabilised me when I was sinking. She challenged me, from a place of deep respect, to excavate beneath the surface and pull out all the hidden critters (emotions, feelings, thoughts, beliefs) that we often hide from the world for fear of us not meeting others' expectations. Brighid has witnessed me at my lowest, sobbing uncontrollably on her floor, wrapped up in a blanket, weeping, shaking – the process of psychosomatic letting go, releasing past pains, old wounds and self-sabotage. She held space for me to unpack 'stuff' that I often didn't want to hear or admit. She made me face my truths, head-on, but always in a loving, compassionate and supportive way. She has been in my corner for over 12 years now. She gave me light when my own light felt extinguished.

The first few months, even years, were spent working on my whole issue around food and my relationship with food. However, I wasn't long into the process when I realised *why* I was eating and acting out in this way. I began to join the dots and see that this was a way to soothe myself, to numb the feelings I didn't want to feel or face. It was my ticket out of pain – or so I thought. I thought food was the enemy, food was the bad guy, food was dangerous and food was my nemesis. But my relationship with food was just a symptom of my disharmonious sense of self. It was highlighting the real issue – that I was a people-pleasing perfectionist, a little girl who was just longing for purpose, passion, meaning, recognition and acknowledgement. This really blew my mind.

I became curious about my habits, thought patterns and internal dialogue – the narratives and stories I played out in my head. I began to read books and do courses on emotional eating, psychological wellbeing, nutritional wellbeing, integrative health coaching, mindfulness, meditation, yoga, energy work, reiki, holistic massage and much more! I dug deep into self-exploration and development. I wanted once and for all to be free from this cage. I no longer wanted to be starved or stuffed; I wanted to be at ease, to be at one with myself. I knew I had a lot of work to do, but I was ready. No more running, no more shaming, no more hiding. I was ready to show up week after week and commit to honouring myself, my needs, my unique journey and, above all, my soul's calling.

Each week, a little voice (my ego) would pop its head up and say, *Maybe you can skip this week* or *You're doing great now, you don't need to go to therapy anymore.* My ego was trying to keep me locked in the past, trapped in the familiar, because the ego wants to keep you safe – but this was 'perceived safety'. For the ego, change is scary and uncertain, so your inner voice will play every trick under the sun to try to stop you from breaking old habits, overcoming addictions and negative behaviours. But we know **that we cannot grow big by thinking small, and we can't mature by staying stuck in the past.**

Why do we hide things from the world? Because we feel we have to uphold a certain image or view in order to feel accepted, valued, and to 'fit in'. We believe the real self, the one that we have barricaded beneath the surface, is not good enough. Even if she whimpered to be expressed or released, we would squeeze her tight or ram sugar down her throat to shut her up. This horrid place, I believe, stems from an internal belief that if the real you were to be let out, it would bring shame upon you, your family or your world.

My personal excavation made me pull my focus away from the external physical world and turn my gaze inwards. I will never forget my first session with Brighid when she said, 'You *can* be free of this,' and I laughed to myself, thinking, *Are you serious?* I genuinely thought I would always use food as my go-to place for comfort when times got tough.

Brighid asked me, 'What would you do or who would you be without this crutch of food? If we took away this habit or this compulsion for food from your life, would you be happy then?' My reaction was, 'No! Oh my goodness, *don't* take this away from me.' Automatically panic and fear set in. Because if this was taken away, what would I do to soothe myself? What would I hide behind? Where would I go? And I realised that the very thing I wanted to be free from was the very thing that I needed to survive. This was a gamechanger for me. I realised that I was subconsciously blocking my own healing because, deep down, I didn't want to let this habit go – it was my anchor.

It has been the greatest journey of my life. It has gifted me internal freedom and lifted the burden of years of pain. It gave me a life that I never thought would be possible. I can proudly say that I'm now out the other side of it. I never in my wildest dreams thought I would ever be free of emotional eating. I thought I'd be caged by this demon for life.

I am forever grateful for this challenge as it has given me more understanding and compassion for other people's journeys. I really believe that in any situation in life, in order to come out the other end of it, you have to first walk through it. Walking through unravels the golden thread, enabling you to meet your emotions, embrace your shadow side and do the self-inquiry work so that, once and for all, you can be liberated.

What is emotional eating?

There are many definitions out there, but I like to keep things simple. Emotional eating is when you eat for reasons other than hunger.

For me, emotional eating is when we eat in unwanted or unwise ways that are driven by unwanted emotions. We are often incapable or unwilling to feel these tough or heavy-hitting emotions because they're too overwhelming, too raw or painful. Emotional eating is a coping mechanism that we use as a way to protect and soothe ourselves when unwanted emotions arise. It is a way to escape reality when times get tough. You might eat because you're bored, tired, stressed, lonely, isolated, scared, sad or angry (which is really sadness in disguise). These underlying emotions then lead to unwanted or superfluous eating patterns in an attempt to quieten the voice within, shun perceived undesirable feelings and ultimately fill the void. However, while food can fill you up, it can never truly fulfil you. I have found time and time again that when people toss the toxic thoughts and shed the stress of shame, it allows them to lose the 'pounds of pain', enabling them to align back to their normal weight.

The why of emotional eating

I believe there are three main things that drive this unwanted way of eating:

1. **Emotional reasons:** Your primary foods are not being fulfilled. The issue is not poor willpower; the issue is often that your inner soul isn't being fulfilled by your deepest desires. Your needs may be suppressed or denied or there may be a lack of emotional awareness and expression. Do a self-enquiry on the four pillars of primary foods to see if anything is out of kilter. If you can fill up your inside world with love and respect, you will be truly nourished, and the need to rely on food to fill you up will lose its potency.

2. **Biochemical, physiological and hormonal imbalances:** If you are constantly living in a stressful state (a sympathetic nervous system dominant state), even though you might know you shouldn't go for the chocolate biscuit at 11am or uncork the bottle of wine at night, succumbing to these temptations becomes almost involuntary. This persistent craving for sugar or glucose-laden foods can be attributed to the body's mistaken belief that it is continuously under threat and in need of immediate energy to combat or escape the perceived danger. Such prolonged exposure to stress signals intensifies the urge for quick energy sources, which impedes rational decision-making when it comes to dietary choices. This causes the biochemistry in your body to change, resulting in these unwanted impulsive eating patterns.

3. **Nutritional depletion:** If there have been years of yo-yo dieting, your body is likely to be lacking essential nutrients, vitamins and minerals. You may have been under-eating or eating diet foods that are often devoid of real nutrients, so deep down at a cellular level you may be starving, which will make you feel hungry all the time. This can lead to food cravings and binges.

The vicious cycle of emotional eating

When it comes to emotional eating, you create a cycle – and it becomes quite a vicious one.

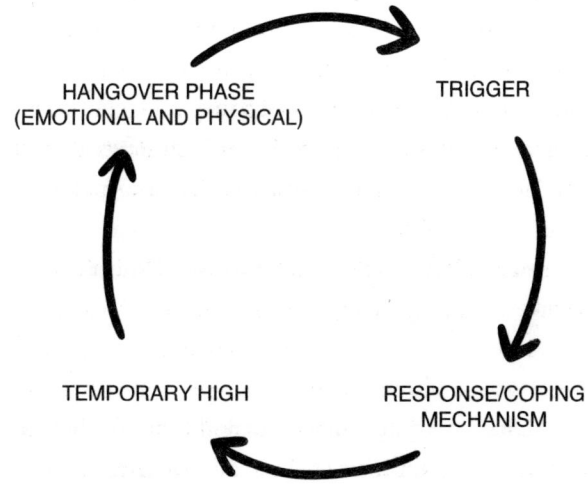

HANGOVER PHASE
(EMOTIONAL AND PHYSICAL)

TRIGGER

TEMPORARY HIGH

RESPONSE/COPING
MECHANISM

1. Trigger

Something in your life opens a wound, unpicks a scar, causing a trigger that elicits an undesired emotional response. For example, a stressful day at work, an argument with a friend, a restless night's sleep might trigger an 'unwanted' or challenging emotion such as anger, sadness, fear, frustration or loneliness.

2. Response/coping mechanism

We then seek out coping mechanisms or distractions to cover up our triggers and numb the unwanted pain. This response or action can be either conscious or unconscious. For many of us, it may manifest as eating with or without awareness, such as devouring a bag of crisps while driving the car, consuming a whole packet of biscuits while watching

TV, finishing a bottle of wine in one sitting or constantly picking at food. How many of us have found ourselves repeatedly returning to the fridge, opening the door and miraculously expecting to find new food that wasn't there five minutes ago?

3. Temporary high – the sugar escape

After step two comes the temporary bliss: the sugar high, the numbing out, the release, the escape, the freedom. While you are in this bliss phase, you forget about what caused you to feel stressed in the first place, but this phase is short-lived and comes with a walloping crash afterwards.

4. The hangover phase

After indulging in a binge-eating session, you are left reeling from a major crash, hitting a slump. You experience a sudden drop in energy levels leading to what is known as the 'hangover phase'. This state can affect you in various ways, either emotionally or physically or both.

The physical aftermath of overeating can be likened to a 'food coma', where your blood sugar levels spike and then plummet, causing a significant drop in mood and energy. You may experience brain fog or feelings of bloating, fullness and general discomfort. Other physical symptoms may also accompany the overwhelming sensation of overeating, such as sweating and headaches, which could lead to feelings of self-judgement, regret, shame and blame.

Emotionally, when the crash comes we get pulled into feelings that can be summarised as FATS:

* **Fear**
* **Anger**

* **Tension**
* **Shame.**

I became aware of the FATS concept many years ago on an Angel Intuitive Course on the east coast of Australia, and it made me realise that these aftermath emotions are the catalysts that keep us trapped in a never-ending cycle.

I believe that fear, the first feeling, is the root emotion, and the others – anger, tension and shame – stem from it.

Healing the wounds, breaking the cycle

It is important to remember that there's no magic pill you can take that will rid you of your stresses, emotions or triggers, nor would we want that. Healing occurs when we meet our emotions with compassion and love and a healthy curiosity to understand why we are feeling this way in the first place. I believe there are valuable lessons to be learned in unpacking our life's journey. It is challenging and painful at times, but excavating to the truth of the matter and exploring the root cause is key to breaking the cycle and becoming free, otherwise we are just putting a Band Aid on it and supressing it.

Apart from reducing stress and filling up on your primary foods, both of which we have spoken about already in detail, there are a few other ways to be free of emotional eating.

Become a detective of the soul

The first step involves awareness and refocus. The healing journey becomes transformative when you shift your viewpoint from diet, food and weight loss to creating inner ease and peace of mind. That is when you begin to change your energy.

Becoming a detective of the soul requires you to ask yourself profound questions such as:

*   What are you truly hungry for in life? (Beyond the plate)

*   What are you craving?

*   You are most likely starving for something – what is it?

I think now, more than ever, as a society we are starved and hungry for more primary foods. Things like more fun, laughter and play. More connection and community, more love, humanity and compassion. What have you potentially restricted or denied yourself in the past that your soul is now calling for?

Take some time to reflect on the questions below. Perhaps even take a few minutes to journal and see what it unearths. Becoming a detective of your relationship with food in an observational, non-judgemental way can be a gateway to commencing and maintaining a healing relationship with food.

*   How do you see or perceive food? Do you see it as healthy? Do you see food as loving and something that will nourish you? Something that will give you energy? Do you view mealtime as a sacred space, a ritual, a blessing, a time to truly connect with yourself and loved ones, a time to be nurtured and nourished?

*   Do you see food as the enemy? The bad guy? Do you view your relationship with food as unloving, destructive and even harmful? Do you dread mealtimes, make excuses around food? Or, conversely, can you not wait for it? Do you have an overriding compulsion or craving that is unstoppable and unnatural? Do you hoover or inhale

food in a forceful or rushed manner, which results in a crumbling recoil and feelings of shame afterwards? Do you think about food all the time? Do you count calories? Are you rigid in your way of eating and your way of thinking around meals? Do you see food as something that needs to be monitored and controlled and restricted?

* Are you indifferent towards food? Does it not bother you? Do you never think about it? Maybe it's not something you have ever really thought about. Perhaps you have a compulsion towards something else instead, such as shopping, smoking, alcohol, stress, exercise or overworking?

For me, this excavation of my relationship with food was a whirlwind, to say the least. When you lift the lid and peek inside, it can be daunting, even terrifying, because you are forced to face, feel and observe all the parts of yourself that you have suppressed or ignored for your entire life.

Self-compassion and acknowledgement

The next pillar to healing and breaking the cycle is a big one – it's to start developing a loving relationship with yourself. Begin by noticing your internal voice: do you speak to yourself in unkind and unloving ways? When we dial down the voice of judgement, dial down the voice of ego, dial down the voice of shame and blame, and instead ramp up the voice of compassion, forgiveness, grace and gratitude – everything changes.

I believe the ultimate medicine when it comes to healing any form of sabotage, internal shaming or blaming and, in particular, emotional eating is self-compassion and deep acknowledgement of your journey.

Deconstruct your emotions

To learn how to recognise your triggers and deconstruct your emotions, I find it useful to break it into four pillars:

* **Observe the emotion:** Don't run away from it. Shine a light on it, invite it in, say hello instead of pushing it down with food or wine. This can be uncomfortable and unpleasant at first, but once you break past this step the healing blooms.

* **Accept the emotion:** Can you accept the emotion without judging it, shaming it or going into self-sabotage mode? This emotion has found a home in your body. It is like a parasite – you can either pretend it's not there and let it get bigger, causing more discomfort and pain, or you can sit with it, close your eyes and scan your body to see where it has taken up residence. Now ask yourself, if this emotion had a name, what would it be? If it had a colour, what would it be? If it held space in an organ or a particular area in your body, where would it be? Is it in your stomach, heart, shoulders or perhaps your head? Then take a few deep breaths and visualise it moving out of your body.

* **Release the emotion:** Find healthy ways to release the emotion.
  » Breathe it out using deep belly breathing (page 55) or the lion's breath (page 40).

  » Talk it out with a trained therapist or a trusted friend or family member.

  » Move it out through exercise and movement.

» Cry it out, as if you are expelling your emotion into the world. If you have a tummy bug and you vomit, you feel better afterwards – the same applies to a good cry.

» Write or draw it out through journalling or expressive art therapy.

✳ **Transform and transmute the emotion:** Every emotion is transient; they ebb and flow. If we go through the steps above we will naturally transform the emotion, and thus create space for a new emotion to be planted instead. Once you've released it, you can fill the space with a new thought, affirmation or mantra. For example, *I love and approve of myself, I accept who I am, I let go of the shame today and I nourish myself in a healthy, loving way.* Once the old negative emotions have been shifted, you can replenish your subconscious mind with positive and transformative thoughts.

Create a gap and be gentle

Create a gap between how you react and the act of your emotional state. Before reaching for the bag of crisps, stop, pause and breathe. Ask yourself, *Am I really hungry for this or am I punishing myself or numbing an emotion?* **When we eat emotionally, it's not that we have a huge hunger for food, it's that we have a huge hunger for life.** Be gentle with yourself on this voyage: be gracious in your journey, be compassionate in your awakenings, be empathetic to your wounded soul, and be grateful for the lessons. Now is your chance to be liberated, to shrug through the mucky departure gates of past shame towards your soul's awakening. Beyond lies a lighter and brighter place, where your heart can be filled with love, your body anchored by a sense of security and your soul set free. Ahead of you lie infinite opportunities.

Gut health

When you feed your gut with healing and sealing foods and beverages, you not only awaken and strengthen your immunity, you also elevate your mental and emotional wellbeing.

Between 75 and 80 per cent of our immune system lies in the gut, so when Hippocrates said 'All disease begins in the gut' he had strong reason for saying so. Gut health is extremely important to our wellbeing, as it is essential to almost every process within the body. It can affect mood, energy, cognition, metabolism, body weight, appetite, immunity and our ability to ward off infection, illness and disease.

Our gut is made up of trillions of bacteria (good and bad) called the microbiome. Ideally, we want more of the good bacteria and less of the bad bacteria. The good bacteria are like a line of defence for our body and our immune system, as they fight off infection and maintain the integrity of the gut lining. However, they are being wiped out more and more by high levels of stress, processed foods, stimulants, artificial sweeteners and a misuse or overuse of medications like anti-biotics, the oral contraceptive pill and some over-the-counter medications.

All of the above can affect the integrity of the gut lining and result in 'leaky gut syndrome', where undigested food particles and toxins seep into the bloodstream. This sends off alarm bells in the body, as these particles are not meant to be there and can be treated as foreign objects, hence the body starts to 'attack' them, which generates an inflammatory response. This is why we are experiencing a rise in autoimmune diseases (such as inflammatory bowel disease, rheumatoid arthritis, psoriasis, etc.).

The gut–brain axis

Have you ever had a 'gut feeling' or butterflies in your stomach? Science is now discovering that these sensations show that your brain and gut are intrinsically connected. The communication system between your gut and brain is called the gut–brain axis (GBA), which refers to the physical and chemical connections between your gut and your brain. Recent studies show that your brain can affect your gut health and your gut can in turn affect your brain health. The gut has often been referred to as the second brain, as many of our powerful neurotransmitters are actually produced in the gut, such as our 'happy hormone' serotonin 5-HT and dopamine. The gut–brain axis connects the gastrointestinal system, the nervous system and the immune system through a vast array of cellular and biochemical messengers throughout the body, including the microbiome, hormones, cytokines and neurotransmitters.

Jay Pasricha, MD, the director of the Johns Hopkins Center for Neurogastroenterology, said, 'Our two brains talk to each other and are in constant communication with one another, so therapies that help one may help the other.' In a way, gastroenterologists (doctors who specialise in digestive conditions) are like counsellors looking for ways to soothe the second brain. If our gut and brain are connected and one can impact the other, then surely the way we treat our gut through our food and lifestyle can impact our immunity, mood and cognitive function.

For many years we thought that the brain sent information to the gut, and it certainly does, but what we didn't realise is that the gut has its own neurons, and that these neurons give the gut an intelligence and awareness of its own.

What might surprise people is that five times more information comes from the gut to the brain than from the brain to the gut. We now know that the health of your gut has a massive impact on how you feel mentally and psychologically. You cannot separate what you think about from how you feel in your gut, so everything you eat has a direct impact on the function and clarity of your brain.

On a deeper level, we must ask ourselves, 'What is my gut telling me?' because the GBA also impacts our spirituality. Sometimes, when we need to make an important decision, we allow the brain and all its noise to speak loudest, ignoring the wisdom of the gut or the whispers from the soul. But decisions can be quite simple: what is your gut instinct telling you or asking of you? In my experience, our deeper, inner wisdom is far better than the voice of the brain, which is a threat-detection system.

A healthy GBA is key if we want to live a life of vitality, health and wellness. So let's think good thoughts, let's visualise good images, let's tell ourselves good stories, because when our brain engages in uplifting stories, it brings vitality to the gut and vice versa. Let's feed the gut nourishing foods, and in return let it feed the brain with positive love and energy.

The gut–brain axis self-enquiry check-in

Below are some questions for you to consider to identify the health of your gut. With a little detective work we can shine a light on whether you need to take steps to improve your gut health – which will lead to a healthier body, a clearer mind and balanced emotions.

After completing the self-enquiry, reflect on your answers and see which areas need the most attention in order to bring balance to your gut and, thus, your mental and emotional wellbeing.

* How often are you bothered by gut symptoms, e.g. bloating, reflux, constipation? These are signals from your gut that something is out of balance and needs a little love and attention.

* Do you take regular medication or over-the-counter drugs? The more OTC or prescribed drugs we take (including the contraceptive pill and antibiotics), the more disruption they will cause to the microbiome in your gut.

* How many different plant-based foods do you eat each week? Include vegetables, fruits, wholegrains, legumes, nuts and seeds (herbs and spices count as a quarter). The aim is to eat 30 different types of these foods each week.

* In an average week, what is your emotional state? How often are you negatively impacted by stress? What areas of your life are causing you most stress? Stress can greatly impact and damage the gut, because when we are stressed blood flows away from the digestive organs to the extremities to protect you and help you enter 'fight or flight' mode.

* How often are you unwell, e.g. with colds and flu? How often you get sick indicates poor gut health, as up to 75 per cent of our immune function is in our gut.

* How many of your meals are home-made? Cooking from scratch leads to healthier eating because you are avoiding processed foods. (Vitamin H = Home cooking!)

* How much of your diet is processed food and beverages? Is lack of time or lack of knowledge driving this?

* How many units of alcohol do you drink per week? Is stress or a lack of joy driving your need for excess or unnecessary alcohol?

* What lifestyle factors do you feel are negatively impacting your gut health? For example, are you always switched on, do you spend a lot of time on screens, do you go to bed too late, overeat or hold on to anger and negative emotions?

* What lifestyle factors do you feel are positively aiding the strength of your immune and gut function? For example, meditation, deep breathing, journalling, talk therapy, exercise, healthy food, good sleep and rest, healthy relationships, a good work–life balance.

How to heal and seal the gut

Maintaining good gut health is essential for overall wellbeing. I find the 'Five Rs' approach useful when it comes to healing and sealing the gut:

* **Remove**
* **Replace**
* **Rebalance/relax**
* **Reinoculate**
* **Repair.**

This process will take time, commitment and perseverance, but it is possible. Please note, however, that if you have any underlying issues, it is always advisable to check with and work alongside your healthcare provider to determine the best approach for your particular situation and symptoms.

Remove

The first step in improving gut health is to remove any potential triggers or irritants that may be causing digestive issues. This can include eliminating certain foods that may be causing inflammation or discomfort, as well as reducing exposure to toxins and pollutants. For example, removing processed foods and artificial additives from your diet can help reduce inflammation in the gut and promote better digestion. If you are experiencing sensitivity, removing some of the most common inflammatory foods such as gluten, dairy and processed sugars can be beneficial. Experiment and see what feels right for you.

Replace

Once potential triggers have been removed, it is important to replace any digestive secretions that your body may be lacking. These might include digestive enzymes, gastric acid and bile acids. (This step may not be necessary.)

I believe it is important to also look at replacing any essential nutrients that may be lacking and contributing to poor digestive health, such as fibre. The gut diversity challenge is a wonderful way to help support the growth of different types of beneficial bacteria in the gut. This challenge encourages participants to consume at least 30 different types of plants (fruits, vegetables, legumes, nuts, seeds, wholegrains, herbs, spices) every week. The greater the diversity, the better your gut health.

Rebalance/relax

Rebalancing the gut microbiome is a vital lifestyle step to healing the gut. This can be achieved by a combination of dietary changes, stress reduction techniques and lifestyle modifications. For example, incorporating stress-reducing activities like yoga, meditation and deep breathing, or creating healthy boundaries and self-care rituals can help rebalance the gut–brain axis and promote better digestion.

Reinoculate

Reinoculation can be done by taking probiotic supplements or consuming foods that are rich in probiotics. For example, adding sources of beneficial bacteria such as natural yogurt, kefir, sauerkraut, kimchi and miso to your diet can help restore a healthy balance of gut microbiota and improve digestion. Prebiotic foods can also play a role in supporting a healthy gut microbiota. Foods such as bananas, onions, garlic and asparagus are all rich sources of prebiotics. (Prebiotics are the food that feed the probiotics – i.e. the good bacteria!)

It is equally important to reinoculate the mind with positive thoughts to support overall health and wellbeing. In order to do this, it is important to engage in activities that promote mental wellbeing, which we will discuss in the Mind section.

Repair

In some cases, the gut may be damaged or inflamed due to various factors like poor diet, stress or medication use. If this is the case, it is important to focus on repairing the gut lining and promoting healing. This can involve adding in supplements like L-glutamine, zinc and collagen to support gut repair and reduce inflammation. Always ask your health practitioner for advice on this.

Reflective exercise to develop a better relationship with your gut

What is your relationship with your gut? Take a few moments to write a letter to your gut. Thank it for all it does. Apologise if you have mistreated it. Begin to reconnect with love and compassion and healthy curiosity to your amazing gut. Notice any resistance or barriers towards this exercise. Offer compassion and forgiveness if there are barriers or blockages.

For years, you might have been told to suck your gut in or hide it away. Now is your chance to reframe this connection and revel in its greatness. Now is the time to start treating it with awe and wonder. By doing this you are not only creating better communication with this area of your body, thus creating less stress in this organ, you are also establishing a new, more loving connection to your body and brain.

This is a powerful exercise in promoting greater gut health. Best of luck. Remember, health begins from the inside out and starts with your willingness and commitment to showing up and honouring yourself with love.

Toolkit for nutritional wellbeing

Eating well will make you feel well.
It's an inside out job.

Nutritional tips

* **Simplify things:** Batch cook meals and freeze so that you're cooking once, eating twice.

* **Increase wholegrains:** Trust me, it's not these types of carbohydrate that have led to the obesity epidemic, it's the processed goods like cakes and white bread. Wholegrains (e.g. brown rice, quinoa, buckwheat) are some of the best sources of nutritional support and provide long-lasting energy.

* **Practise home cooking** (also known as vitamin H): It's a fundamental step to healthier living. When you make your own meals you know what's going into them – and they don't need a long list of ingredients or to take hours to prepare.

* **Drink enough water:** Hydration not only impacts our inner health and vitality, it's also important for our external glow and sparkle. In today's world, many of us are living in a state of chronic or mild dehydration. If you are experiencing lack of concentration or focus, irritability, decreased cognitive function, aches and pains, dull, lifeless and dreary skin and eyes, or you are experiencing constant fatigue and tiredness, you might just be suffering from mild or chronic dehydration. When we think of a well-hydrated body, we can imagine the cells resemble a fresh, firm, plump, round grape. Unfortunately, when we get dehydrated, that grape shrinks down and becomes shrivelled like a raisin. In the mind, dehydration can feel similar – you might experience feelings of being withered and dried up. The best way to check your hydration is to become aware of the colour of your urine. If your urine is dark yellow, it is a sign that you are dehydrated and need to drink more water. If it's too clear, it's a sign that you may be drinking too much water. This isn't great either as you could be putting extra pressure on your kidneys and bladder, which can flush out essential electrolytes from the body. The ideal colour of your urine should be a pale, straw-yellow colour. The suggested daily water intake is 1.5–2 litres per day. Generally, the more active you are, the more water you should drink. Keep a bottle with you at all times to encourage sipping throughout the day (in your car, in your handbag, on your desk), Add lemon, mint or

berries to your water to add variety and set reminders on your phone to remind you to drink.

* **Increase sweet vegetables:** Naturally sweet vegetables (e.g. sweet potato, beets, carrots, butternut squash) are the perfect medicine for the sweet tooth. Instead of depending on processed sugar, you can add more naturally sweet flavours to your diet and dramatically reduce sugar cravings.

* **Increase leafy green vegetables:** These are essential for creating long-lasting health. They are packed with phytonutrients and help to alkalise the body and cleanse the blood. More specifically, they help to detoxify the body and improve liver, gallbladder and kidney function.

* **Crowd out:** Eat less sugar and processed foods; consume less coffee, alcohol and tobacco. Eat more vegetables, fruits, wholegrains and drink more water. Add more meditation, exercise, sleep. Eventually, you will naturally crowd out processed foods, sitting on the couch, fatigue and low mood.

* **Drink hot water and lemon** (or ginger tea) first thing in the morning (ideally 30 minutes before eating) or before meals to help your digestion. This will help stimulate your liver and bowels and acts as a powerful cleansing process for the body.

* **Buy local and eat in season:** Eating in season and locally is not only a sustainable practice, it ensures the freshest and most flavourful produce while promoting variety and diversity in our diet. It is a small but impactful way to

support our health, immunity, community and environment.

* **Bless your food:** Saying grace before meals is a powerful way to make mealtime a sacred space. Take a moment to be grateful for the hands that made and prepared the food and for the blessings this food will bring to your body. With each bite you will be reminded of the abundance and love that surround you. Take a moment to thank every cell in your body, particularly your digestive organs, for all that they will do to assimilate this food so that you can be truly nourished.

* **Go back to basics:** Avoid ultra-processed foods as much as possible and eat the rainbow instead (see page 142).

* **Increase fibre:** Fibre is essential for gut health and for the health of good bacteria in the gut. It helps to regulate digestion, maintain a healthy weight and reduce the risk of some chronic diseases, such as diabetes and heart disease.

* **Reduce blood sugar spikes:** When blood sugar levels spike the body releases insulin to help regulate it, but consistently high levels of insulin can lead to insulin resistance and increase the risk of developing type 2 diabetes. Additionally, frequent spikes in your blood sugar levels can contribute to other alarming factors such as inflammation, weight gain and increased risk of cardiovascular disease. By eating a balanced diet rich in fibre, healthy fats and lean protein, as well as lifestyle habits such as staying active and managing stress, you can help stabilise your blood sugar levels. Prioritising a diet that's

low in refined sugars and carbohydrates can also help prevent blood sugar spikes and promote overall health and wellbeing.

* **Eat mindfully:** Slow down and chew your food.

Foods to help rebalance the nervous system

* **Magnesium-rich foods:** Magnesium is the 'relaxing' mineral and can be found in dark chocolate, avocados, legumes, nuts, seeds, wholegrains, leafy greens, bananas, cacao and oily fish.

* **Foods high in B vitamins:** These help to keep your nerves healthy. They include lean meats, dairy products, eggs, leafy green vegetables, wholegrains, nuts, seeds and legumes.

* **Antioxidant-rich foods:** Antioxidants are compounds that help protect the body from damage caused by free radicals, which are unstable molecules that can harm cells and contribute to inflammation, premature ageing and various diseases. Antioxidants are powerful agents that neutralise these free radicals, thereby reducing oxidative stress in the body. Foods that are high in antioxidants include colourful fruits and vegetables such as berries and dark green leafy vegetables, nuts and seeds, herbs and spices such as turmeric, cinnamon and ginger, and good-quality dark chocolate and green tea.

* **Anti-inflammatory diet:** Include healthy fats in your diet such as omega-3 fatty acids found in fish, flax seeds, olive oil, avocados and walnuts, which have anti-inflammatory properties. Choose whole, unprocessed foods whenever

possible as they're typically lower in inflammatory compounds, and incorporate herbs and spices like turmeric, ginger and cinnamon into your meals.

* **Reduce stimulants:** Caffeine acts on the adrenal glands by stimulating the production of adrenaline. When adrenaline is released, your blood sugars elevate to provide more energy and your digestion is affected as blood races to your extremities to activate fight or flight.

Good nutrition is key to nourishing your body, fuelling your mind and balancing your nervous system.

Light-up moments

Light-up moments are those special occasions when something seemingly ordinary or mundane suddenly becomes extraordinary and fills us with joy, excitement, hope or inspiration. These moments of light bring us back to our centre, ground us and enable us to feel grace and gratitude. These glimmer or sparkle moments allow our nervous system to regulate, our heart to open and our soul to expand. They change us chemically and hormonally; they shift us emotionally, bringing more joy into our hearts; socially, they enable us to open, connect and engage; and spiritually they enable us to expand our consciousness, awaken to our truths and align to our values.

It's important to pay attention to and appreciate these light-up moments, as they can bring happiness, gratitude and a renewed sense of wonder to our lives. They serve as reminders to slow down, be present and find joy in the little things.

Hopefully, as you apply the tips in this chapter you'll start noticing more simple moments that light up your life.

Light-up moments for the body

◊ Enjoying a delicious meal

◊ A perfect warm cup of tea

◊ The feel-good 'endorphin high' after a great workout

◊ The serenity and calmness that arises during savasana at the end of a yoga class

◊ Dancing like no one is watching and letting yourself be free

◊ A good night's sleep

◊ The freshness and sense of invigoration you feel after a beautiful walk in nature

◊ The feeling of wholesomeness and rejuvenation when you nourish your body with nutritious foods and beverages that are supportive to your immune system

◊ Getting into flow state when playing your favourite sports, whether golf, tennis, football, or going for a hike or cycle

◊ The sense of peace and ease you feel after engaging in deep-breathing exercises

◊ Taking a refreshing shower or bath after a long day

◊ Snuggling up in a cosy blanket and feeling completely relaxed and content.

MIND

The words we use and the thoughts we think shape and create the lives we live, the people we become and the health and happiness we obtain.

CHAPTER 5

AWAKENING
THE MIND

When you think about your wellbeing, do you think about the connection between your mind and your physical wellbeing, or do you think about your health only in terms of physicality? In the world of wellness, I fear there is still an overemphasis on building physical health, with disregard, avoidance or simply not enough knowledge around how to build, maintain and manage our mental fitness. Of course, exercise, nutrition and sleep are super important, as we discussed in the Body section, but without tending to our precious minds, we will never be fully healed and whole.

Just as we exercise our body to improve our physical fitness, we need to exercise our mind to improve our mental fitness.

Becoming aware of my inner dialogue and my self-talk patterns was gamechanging for me. I became aware that I had a tendency to doubt myself, judge myself, be a little harsh on and critical of myself. I would dim my lights and see myself as a victim of circumstance. I would regularly blame and berate myself for not being good enough, which held me back and prevented me from taking certain opportunities. However, as I began to delve into personal development, I started to realise the power of my own thoughts and beliefs. I learned that the stories I told myself about who I was and what I was capable of greatly influenced my reality. It was a difficult process to confront and change these narratives. I'm still a work in progress, as I believe we all are. But I knew that in order to truly live a fulfilling life, I had to start changing the dialogue within. In this section, as I share the 11 pillars of building mental fitness, I hope to inspire and empower you to do the same. I believe that focusing on our internal mental fitness and becoming aware of our inner stories can truly change our lives for the better.

During my pharmacy training, the primary focus was on the physical body. As part of our education, we studied anatomy, which involved working with cadavers (bodies donated to science). While studying this was very important, it also triggered a realisation. I experienced an awakening as I reflected on the stark reality that when observing a deceased body, all the signs of life have departed. There is no energy present, no emotion racing, no feelings being felt, no thoughts, no spirit – nothing. What remains is the physical shell, devoid of the essence that once animated it. I've always been fascinated by how truly interlinked the mind and body are, and this realisation prompted a deeper exploration of the rich tapestry of interconnectedness between the physical, mental and spiritual aspects of human existence. I realised that there are certain limitations in modern Western medicine, as it often neglects the holistic essence that underlies healing. One of the pillars of health and wellbeing lies in the level of ease, peace and grace we hold in our mind, for it directly impacts all other aspects of our lives. Indeed, the benefits of developing mental fitness are vast. You will achieve:

* Greater inner ease and peace

* Increased clarity and focus

* More space in the mind

* Greater cognitive function, e.g. enhanced memory, concentration and problem-solving skills

* Reduced stress and anxiety

* Increased resilience in the face of adversity

* Enhanced creativity and innovation

* Better emotional intelligence, leading to healthier relationships with others and with yourself

* Greater self-awareness

* More loving and supportive self-talk.

Our thoughts become our internal chemistry: the mind–body connection

I learned this concept from the scientist, doctor and author Dr Bruce Lipton, who has revolutionised our understanding of how our beliefs and thoughts shape our biology. He is a biologist known for excavating the role of epigenetics in shaping our health and behaviour. Epigenetics is the study of how genes can be turned on or off without changing the actual DNA sequence. 'Epi' means above or on top of, so 'epigenetics' refers to changes in gene expression (when genes are turned on or off) that occur on top of the DNA sequence itself. These changes can be influenced by various factors in our environment, such as our lifestyle choices and emotional experiences.

It used to be thought that our genes are our destiny, so whatever we inherit is ultimately going to become our fate. However, we are now learning through the science of epigenetics that this is untrue. When you are born your genes are inherited, which is like you've been handed a loaded gun; but what pulls the trigger is dependent on the lifestyle that you live. The trigger either turns on certain genes that can express in certain ways or turns off certain genes, preventing them expressing in certain ways.

Environmental factors such as stress, emotions and diet can influence gene expression and the development of cells and organisms. Imagine that every single cell in your body has a pair of ears, and every single cell is receptive. So, each cell can hear every thought that you think, and it can feel every emotion that you feel. Each cell will then react and respond, or switch on or off, according to the signals that they've been sent from your thoughts and your emotions.

When you wake up, when the alarm goes off, what do you think about? Do you think positively and in a self-nourishing way? Or do you have a tendency to be negative and go into a stressed state? Do you find yourself having thoughts of dismay at the prospect of facing yet another day? Perhaps the antici-pation of heavy traffic ahead or the overwhelming feeling of having a multitude of tasks awaiting your attention feeds your mind. While these anxious thoughts are *common*, they are not necessarily *normal*. They are not normal over prolonged periods of time, not normal for the health of our nervous system, and not normal for the functioning of each cell in our bodies.

The language we use in our minds becomes the food that nourishes our cells. The vibrational frequency of the words becomes the beverage they drink, and the dispelled energy from these feelings, emotions and thoughts becomes our cells' home environment, from which they either dance and radiate or wilt and shrink.

Our cells will react to whatever frequency or energy is created in our minds. This is mind-blowing! Hence, if we are thinking negative thoughts, we will be sending out distress signals, creating a stressful environment for our cells to live in. Their environment thus then becomes one of stress and strain. On the flip side, if we can become more aware of our thoughts, more aware of the way we're communicating to ourselves, we can change this, and so we can change our chemistry and the activation or deactivation of our gene expressions. Take, for example, two plants in a garden. One plant is nurtured daily with love, care and positive words; the other plant is neglected and overlooked. The nurtured plant goes on to blossom and flourish while the other wilts and withers. In the same way, words carry power and thoughts can transform.

Applying this idea to our own lives, by thinking more compassionately, by sending more love to our bodies, by being kinder to ourselves, we can change our internal chemistry and create more internal harmony and ease.

To understand the power of the mind–body connection in a more tangible way, think of when something difficult happens in your life and you feel sad. This feeling of sadness has been generated by a thought. As a result of this feeling, your body starts to produce tears and you cry. As a result of a thought, you have physically produced tears. Similarly, when you feel embarrassed or ashamed your cheeks go bright red. This is a physical response triggered by an emotion. In situations of embarrassment or heightened emotion, the body's fight or flight response can be activated, leading to increased blood flow and the dilation of blood vessels, which results in the reddening of the skin – a visible manifestation of the person's emotional state. This physical reaction is involuntary and a clear example of how our emotions and thoughts can directly influence our physiological responses through the mind–body connection.

Ego versus essence

As an integrative health coach, I am continually reminded of the delicate dance between ego and essence in our lives. The ego is the part of us that is driven by fear, insecurity and the need for validation from others. It is the part of us that fears being left behind, dreads separation and isolation, and hates change. It would much prefer to stay stuck somewhere that is unloving, unkind and even destructive because it is familiar, rather than have to change or start anew because this change is too overwhelming – to the ego it is far too scary and unsafe. The ego has a bad reputation – people believe the ego is toxic, wrong, even dangerous – but deep down, like any villain, the ego is just lost, scared and afraid. It actually loves you, but it has a funny way of showing it! It will try to cajole you away from any situation that it perceives is unsafe, even if that situation is a new opportunity. But rather than resist or hate it, we must learn to tame the ego, for it is part of our existence. If we hate any part of ourselves, we will never be fully whole and healed. **The only way we can heal and become at ease is if we compassionately use love as our guiding star, not resistance as our navigator.**

We must recognise the non-serving part of the ego but not suppress it; any form of suppression leads to depression, causing an internal tug of war and a lack of ease within. Despite the ego being the voice in our heads that often tells us we are not good enough, not smart enough, not worthy of love and success, despite it being the part of us that seeks to control, manipulate and dominate others, we must turn the lens in a different direction and seek to find out why the ego might be doing this *for* us instead of why it is doing it *to* us.

Now that we know why the ego acts the way it does, does this mean we have to honour its callings and obey its messages? Absolutely not. We can listen with a healthy curiosity, but we have a choice as to which callings we follow – the ego or the essence. The ego is like a toddler throwing a tantrum: it demands attention, validation and control, just like a child throwing a fit in the middle of a store. It screams for what it wants, regardless of the consequences or the impact on others. But just like with a child having a meltdown, giving in to the ego's demands is not the best course of action. While it may temporarily quiet the screaming, it will only reinforce the behaviour and lead to more tantrums in the future.

Instead, like a responsible parent, we must set boundaries in a loving way and take control of the situation. We don't neglect, ignore or deny its callings: we listen, but then we guide it towards a healthier, more balanced way of being by tuning into the voice of our inner essence, which I believe is the calling of the guiding heart.

What is our essence? It is our true nature, the authentic self that is connected to higher source energy. It is the part of us that is pure, true, loving, compassionate and kind. Think of a new baby when they are born. They are pure, mesmerising, charismatic, loving. This essence is still within us all. It is just that as we navigate through life, this purity can get drowned out or 'polluted' by the external world. But this inner essence is still within us all.

It is the part of us that feels at home, at ease, and brings relief, acceptance and permission to just be yourself. It is the part of us that is driven by a sense of humanity, purpose, passion and connection to something greater than ourselves. Our essence is a loving voice that never uses the word *should*. It uses *could* or *will*, as it breeds enthusiasm, motivation and optimism, not the negativity and shame that often stems from the egoic voice. If we allow our ego to dominate our thoughts and actions, we become disconnected from our essence.

How do we know the difference between the voice of ego and the voice of essence?

These two voices are derived from two very different emotions: the ego voice stems from fear, while the essence voice stems from love. They both carry a different frequency, a different pace, a different rhythm. The voice of the ego is fast-paced, urgent, chaotic, disorganised and frantic. Fear breeds spin-off emotions like anger, frustration, comparison, judgement, shame and blame. Fear is the main emotion of the ego.

In contrast, the voice of the essence stems from a deep-seated place of love or divine grace. This emotion breeds spin-off energies of compassion, empathy, understanding, forgiveness, joy, ease and grace. Its rhythm and pace is very different from the ego's. The essence feels calm, grounded and solid. There's strength, stillness and solitude to it; it's not in a rush, it's not chaotic, busy or frantic. It is loving, caring and stable.

The ego screams from the head, while the essence leans from the heart. Over time, you will get to know these different voices. In order to learn how to decipher between these two voices, you must initially allow yourself time and space in silence, stillness, solitude and nature so that you can really tune in. You must reduce the noise and the distraction of the ego and allow yourself to drop into the spaciousness of the soul, where you can hear, feel and know the voice of your essence. It will communicate to you through gentle whispers, bodily sensations, inner visions or images or via intuition.

During a retreat I hosted, a client came seeking clarity and direction in her life. Throughout the retreat, she struggled to let go of her ego's voice, which often told her she was not capable of making significant changes or following her dreams. This inner critic made her doubt her worth and potential, leading to feelings of insecurity and fear. However, as the retreat progressed, she began to connect with her essence through meditation, introspection and soul-connecting activities. She realised that, deep down, she had a strong desire to move abroad, as she was not feeling aligned or fulfilled in her current environment. Something was telling her or nudging her to move. At the time she didn't really know why, but despite her ego's attempts to hold her back, she decided to lean in, listen and follow this call.

She took the leap of faith and relocated to a new space. Not long after relocating, she met the man of her dreams and fell in love. Her whole world transformed in ways beyond her wildest dreams. She not only found love but also a new sense of freedom, adventure and fulfilment. By listening and connecting to her essence, it changed her life for the better.

Ultimately, the journey from ego to essence is a lifelong process of self-discovery and self-acceptance. It requires courage, resilience, patience, trust and a willingness to confront the parts of ourselves that we may not always like or understand. But it is through this journey that we are able to cultivate a sense of inner peace, joy and fulfilment that transcends the limitations of our ego and allows us to live a life that is truly aligned with our highest potential.

CHAPTER 6

THE 11 PILLARS OF BUILDING MENTAL FITNESS

Now that we know the importance of our mind and its impact on our bodies, what can we do to build mental fitness? There are 11 pillars to help create, build and maintain greater mental strength and internal fitness of the mind:

1. Journalling – pen, paper, power!

2. Meditation – going beyond the noise

3. Mirror work – self-love and relationship to self

4. Visualisation – design your destiny

5. Breaking through limited beliefs and habits and shifting out of subconscious programs

6. Self-talk – the stories we tell ourselves and the art of reframing

7. Affirmations – declarations for life

8. Re-centring routines that trigger positive transformation

9. Forgiveness – rest for the mind, liberation for the soul

10. Gratitude – unlocking the power of grace

11. Nutrition, hydration and gut health.

1. Journalling – exploring the mind through writing

Many of us might think journalling is 'just writing', but it is so much more. Journalling is an exploration of the mind through writing. It is the act of writing down your feelings, emotions and thoughts as a way to process, express and release them. It is a powerful tool for self-reflection, stress relief and personal growth, and is in itself a form of mindfulness and meditation. In yoga, the breath is the gateway to the soul. Well, believe it or not, journalling is another tool we can use to dig deeper into our soul, come home to our heart and understand all the corners of our subconscious mind. I believe it truly acts as a beautiful tool to awaken and cleanse our mind.

Journalling is essential for excavating the mind; it allows you to explore all the hidden or unseen thoughts that only come to light when we start to write. The art of writing illuminates the subconscious mind and the programs that it is running. It allows us to see, observe and keep a check on where our shadow is rising. Just like watching a movie, themes become apparent, the script becomes clear, your character becomes obvious. Do you play the villain or the victim? Journalling gifts you the opportunity to receive some lightbulb moments, then press pause. You can then observe what's happening, 'pull it out' gently and gradually, like a thread, so that you don't untangle the whole thing at once. The more you journal, the more you can gently pull at this piece of thread, rub it between your fingers and ask, *What is actually going on in my life? What am I actually doing? How am I actually showing up? Is this serving me or spoiling me? Is it healing me or hurting me?*

Benefits of journalling

Your own personal bible

When you start to journal, you begin to observe your thoughts, feelings, reactions and actions, and shine a light on your daily behaviours. It becomes your own story. This 'bible' serves as a great guidance tool: just as people turn to literature or scripture for inspiration, you can revisit your past entries and reflect on the lessons you've learned. You will see how much you have grown and find guidance for navigating current challenges and decisions in your life.

Your safety net

Your journal can act almost as a comfort or a soother, a place where you can truly be yourself, express the deepest essence of everything that resides within you, without fear or shame, without anyone watching, listening, hearing or judging. It acts as a safe haven for you to drop down, release, relax and let the heaviness of the day or any burdens you have been shouldering be released and set free.

Bring order to the chaos

Some mornings, when you wake up, you might feel that you have too many plates spinning (*I never rang that person back, I didn't reply to that text message or email, I have to order books for the kids*). This can be exhausting, stressful and damaging for your mental health. Journalling is a magic tool to reveal this chaos or busyness in the mind. By taking some time to pause, make a list and articulate your thoughts, you can bring structure, formality and clarity to the whirlwind.

Reveal the shadow

Journalling is a fascinating way to reveal the light and unearth the shadow within. It highlights things that we have a tendency to run away from: a thought pattern, an action, reaction or behaviour type. Journalling allows you to be honest with yourself in a non-threatening way. And giving ourselves time and space to be truthful, to really open up, generates immense freedom. Journalling was a potent gateway for me personally to meet my shadow, to meet the parts of me that I perceived to be flawed and untangle all the nonsense that I no longer needed.

The vortex

Just like a vortex, journalling can create a distance, a gap between you and your thoughts. This can help you view your thoughts from a more objective perspective, allowing you to grace yourself with compassion and reverence. It also grants permission for speech, expression and freedom without the repercussions that we sometimes fear when we speak our truths in the outer world.

Cultivate confidence

Just as journalling reveals the shadow, it can also shine a light on the wonderful parts of ourselves, allowing us to generate gratitude and confidence for all the wonderful things we have accomplished. Documenting these successes enables the development of greater self-trust, inner love and confidence.

Reduce mental anxiety and stress

Journalling is a form of brain dump, a safe space for you to write down your worries, fears and stresses. Externalising them makes them feel more manageable and it's also a form of self-care. Journalling is, I believe, a form of meditation. It's mindfulness in motion. Mindfulness is when you become aware of the present moment unfolding right before you without judgement, shame or comparison. When you journal, whatever comes up for you, the key is not to judge the thoughts, no matter how dark they get. Let go of the need to control, and simply allow it to be. Then you release it. You shed it from the mind. This helps reduces strain and stress within the nervous system.

Physical and emotional wellbeing

The biggest reason why journalling has a positive impact on our physical health is because it reduces anxiety and stress, reducing stress hormones and taking the body out of sympathetic-dominant state. This allows the nervous system to regulate. **By reducing conflict in the mind, you reduce strain on the body.**

Types of journalling

One size doesn't fit all. There is no one right or wrong way to journal, and often you will create your own avenue for expression. There are different methods of journalling, but you might find a blend of styles suits you. For example, you could start off by writing a list of tasks and then reflect on your thoughts and emotions by journalling in a more stream-of-consciousness way. To get you going, here are the main methods of journalling. Give them a try and see which is the best fit for you.

Proprioceptive writing

'Proprio' comes from the Latin word 'oneself', so this method focuses on a journey into your mind and soul. You write about your thoughts, feelings, actions and behaviours. It is a conscious stream of writing. You can literally just write whatever is in your mind. Just throw it all down, there's nothing you can't write. This way, you're allowing yourself to hear the inner voice and explore your psyche.

Morning pages

This journalling technique was described by Julia Cameron in her book *The Artist's Way*. It involves writing three pages of stream-of-consciousness, uncensored thoughts first thing in the morning. You empty your mind onto the page without worrying about spelling, grammar, coherence or even logic. The goal of the morning pages is to wipe your mind clear of any mental clutter or dark debris, tap into your creativity, uncover underlying issues that may be bubbling up to the surface and at risk of influencing your day-to-day decisions and behaviours. By engaging in this powerful daily writing practice, you remove any creative blocks, release anxiety and pent-up emotions, and gain valuable insights for the day ahead. Just pick up a pen and write anything down. Don't worry about what will come out. If you feel stuck, just write 'I feel stuck and I don't know what to write', and keep writing until the floodgates open.

Reflective journalling or prompted journalling

This technique involves writing about your thoughts, feelings and experiences in a reflective way. It typically involves looking back at your day, a specific event or period of time in your life and writing about what happened, how you felt and what you learned from the experience. Prompted journalling involves using specific questions that trigger you to unearth the deepest essence of what lies within you. These prompts can be specific questions or open-ended statements which are designed to spark introspection. They draw your attention to topics you may not have considered on your own, supporting you to evolve and become the greatest version of yourself.

Some examples of prompted journalling questions include:

* How would I like to show up for myself today?

* What are the qualities that I would like to display to the world today?

* If I could write a letter to my teenage self, what's the one piece of advice I'd give them?

* If my body could talk to me right now, what would it tell me or what would it ask of me?

* If my soul could speak to me right now, what advice would it give me or what would it ask of me? What is the message it is trying to send me today?

* What went well for me today? What am I grateful for?

* What potentially didn't serve me today? What would I like to let go of?

* Where did I show up for a friend or family member today or this week? How do I show compassion? How do I show kindness?

* How can I show that compassion and kindness to myself today, tomorrow or this week?

These are very simple questions, but when you think about them and dig deeper into the mind, they can provide powerful answers.

Prioritised journalling

This type of journalling involves writing lists or developing your own CODE: Calendar Of Daily Events. Your calendar of daily events becomes your non-negotiable list of things to complete. When you write them down, you spring them into the universal energy field, helping you to commit to them and manifest the outcomes. For example, you can write down one thing you can do today to nourish your mind (meditate, get fresh air, affirmations), one thing that will nourish your body (have a green juice, go for a walk or do some yoga), and one thing that will nourish your soul (meet up with a friend, read a few pages of an inspirational book, do something you're passionate about). These may appear to be small things, but when done regularly, they are in fact the big things that lead to the greatest transformations.

Gratitude journalling

This involves simply writing down things that you're grateful for. The list doesn't have to be long; the key is to rotate the things you are thankful for daily so you're not writing down the same things repeatedly. Be sure to write down small things, not just big things, because the greater the emphasis on the smaller wins, the more beauty, pleasure and joy you can extract from everyday activities. This way you won't be waiting for the weekend or that holiday to bring you happiness.

Setting yourself up for success: the do's and don'ts

* **There's no right or wrong.** So just do it. Don't try to analyse it, and if you are analysing it, just write that. It doesn't have to be perfect. It can be as messy, as scribbly and as scrappy as you want. It's not something that has to be displayed to the world.

* **Release the attachment to the negativity.** When you start to write, especially in the morning pages, you might find it's all negative: *I'm really tired* or *I slept crap and I have to go into a big meeting today*. But the truth is, if you don't write it, it's going to stick in your mind and affect your energy, and that energy is going to manifest in your life. By writing it out, you can dispel and release that negativity.

* **Make it your own sacred space.** Find a space in the house just like you would do with a meditation, maybe light a candle, put on some relaxing music, and set yourself up. This can be a precious mindful moment. You might also like to add some motivational pictures to your journal (a picture of your family, a blue sky, the ocean) or a mantra, so your journal becomes an inspirational vision board or toolkit.

* **Don't censor yourself.** Don't be hard on yourself. Remember that journalling is a mental process and it's okay to have ups and downs and breaks in your practice. Be kind to yourself as you explore your emotional world.

2. Meditation – the magical portal to greater mental fitness and internal peace

I could write an entire book on meditation alone, but I will just share the key points of why meditation is an incredible way of clearing and calming the mind and creating inner ease.

To put it simply, meditation is the journey inward. It's the soft landing into your heart, an arrival home into your essence and a departure towards greater freedom and wisdom. It opens the gates to an inner world that is beyond reasoning or intellect, sometimes even beyond comprehension. It resonates with a deep knowingness, an undercurrent of simplicity in its own right. Meditation drills down through the layers of unwanted emotions, sensations or information stored within. Moving past these layers of armour, you arrive at an inner well of peace, tranquillity and love. I believe meditation is the ultimate gateway home, to the place of peace that resides within all of us. The journey to this inner sanctuary may be different for everyone, depending upon our 'layers', past experiences, levels of trauma or inner turmoil. Some of these layers can bring up significant feelings, which might be challenging, so make sure you practice in a space where you feel safe, and if you find it overwhelming, pause and seek professional support from a therapist. Nonetheless, with daily practice and a commitment to move past these uncomfortable sensations, you can land softly into your soul's place of deep rest, restoration and contemplation. Your home.

Meditation helps burn away the ego's frantic voice of fear

When we meditate, we literally emit different brain waves. We receive information at a much deeper level than we do during normal consciousness. When we build meditation into our daily lives, we emanate more positive and authentic vibes. Although invisible, they carry an energy. When we tune into our higher self during meditation, we begin to reconnect with our essence.

Meditation helps us become aware of our thoughts and enables us to wisely choose which ones we give more energy to. Energy flows where our thoughts go. As a result, we can see our world differently. It becomes a kinder, more accepting place when we choose to see love instead of anger and peace instead of hatred.

Lifting the fog

I'm sure many of us have experienced that feeling of being foggy or blocked in our mind. Perhaps too many to-do lists, too many stressors pulling at you, having to constantly be 'on', absorbing the world of social media, other people's thoughts, opinions and judgements! *It's a lot.* And this noise causes our mind to feel like it's being bombarded 24/7, so much so that you can't think clearly, you can't switch off at night, which impacts your sleep, and it even causes you to think differently, propelling you into stress mode and making you a little crazy and unrecognisable.

Meditation helps to calm this noise and clear the chaos so we can think more clearly, perform better, be more compassionate to others and ourselves, and live with more ease.

You're not meant to stop the thoughts!

When you start to meditate, it can highlight all the noise that's going on in your mind. It might even feel as if the noise has suddenly been amplified, you've turned up the radio and your head is going to explode! This was a revelation for me. I realised that it wasn't that the volume was being turned up; rather, the noise was already in my mind – I had just paused long enough to become aware of it. Once you have awareness, you can change things. Rather than your mind ruling you, you can now take control of your mind.

This might seem a little daunting at the start. People often feel uncomfortable hearing their thoughts. However, it does become easier and the benefits are unbelievable. The important thing to remember is that you're not meant to stop thinking during meditation. So many people say to me, *I can't do it, it's not working, my mind is too busy, I can't stop thinking!* This is normal. You are not meant to stop thinking – if you stopped thinking you would be dead! The aim is to become aware of your thoughts and then slowly detach from them and let them go. Meditation is like watching clouds passing in your mind. You become aware of the thought, say hello to it, welcome it (even if it's a negative or an unloving thought), and then let it move on with ease and grace. Each time these thoughts come, which they inevitably will, the art of meditation brings you back to a focal point, such as your breath or a mantra. This refocused concentration brings you into the present moment, into your heart, which is love, and away from the busyness of the mind, which is fear.

Benefits of meditation

* **Reduced stress and anxiety:** Meditation affects the nervous system by taking you out of the reactive stressful states, enabling you to enter a flow state, ultimately calming the mind and relaxing the body.

* **Improved focus and concentration:** It trains the concentration part of the brain by bringing you back to a focal point when your mind wanders. This enhances cognitive function, improves concentration and memory and increases mental clarity.

* **Changes to brain wave activity:** Whether you're in a deep sleep, giving a presentation or taking a test, your brain is abuzz with activity. We can see this activity reflected in our brain waves. Meditation helps us move from the gamma or beta brain waves of activity and alertness to alpha and theta brain waves of deep relaxation and visualisation.

* **Increased self-awareness and greater emotional well-being:** As meditation helps you to become more aware of your thoughts, feelings and bodily sensations, you develop a greater sense of self-awareness and introspection. It also helps to regulate emotions and promote a positive mindset.

* **Enhanced restoration and sleep:** Meditation can help to improve sleep quality by calming the mind and relaxing the body, making it easier to fall asleep and stay asleep throughout the night.

* **Greater mental health and reduced symptoms of depression:** Studies have shown that regular meditation practice can help to alleviate symptoms of depression and improve overall mental health.

* **Lower blood pressure:** Meditation has been shown to reduce blood pressure and improve cardiovascular health by promoting relaxation and reducing stress.

* **Enhanced creativity:** Meditation can enhance creativity and innovative thinking by quieting the mind, reducing distractions and fostering a sense of openness and receptivity.

* **Improved connection and relationships:** Meditation can help to cultivate compassion, empathy and a deeper connection with others, leading to healthier and more fulfilling relationships.

* **Present moment awareness:** Mindfulness meditative practices and breath-focused awareness pull us away from distraction and racing thoughts, anchoring us in the here and now so we can fully experience the present moment.

Types of meditation

Each type of meditation has its own unique benefits and practices. It's important to explore the different types of meditation to find out what works best for you and your individual needs. It's about finding a method that suits you depending on what stage of life you are in. When I was studying yoga psychology with Ashley Turner in Los Angeles, she simplified the various types of meditation by putting them into two categories:

1. Formal

2. Informal

Each of these categories has several subtypes. Please note: I have added my own interpretations and explanations of meditation from what I have learned over the years. I have woven my own life experiences with the learnings from yoga psychology training, which I hope explains in a simple way what meditation is, how you do it and how you can incorporate it into your daily life.

1. Formal

These are the types of practice you might picture in your mind when you think of meditation. They involve setting aside 10 to 20 minutes to sit down in solitude and meditate.

Solitude meditation

This meditative practice involves finding peace and stillness by distancing yourself from the distractions of daily noise. It is a practice of seeking inner tranquillity and clarity through quiet contemplation and reflection. You can use meditation aids such as timed bells, mala beads, connecting with the divine light of higher consciousness, connecting with your angels or past loved ones, or simply focus on anchoring yourself into the earth for security, safety and solitude.

Sadhana is another form of solitude meditation; it is a disciplined daily practice that includes silence, meditation, breathwork, yoga, chanting or other spiritual practices to start the day with focus and mindfulness. Essentially it means setting aside some time each morning in silence to cultivate a deeper connection to the self, to clear the mind and to gain clarity, safety and love.

Concentration (focused meditation)

Concentration or focused meditative practices are like a dam for the mind. Just as a dam blocks the water, this meditation practice helps block the noise and the busyness of the mind. It loosens your attachment to distractions and addictions. It involves having a pointed focus on something, for example:

* Breath-focused meditation

* Body-scan meditation

* Mantra (mind tool) meditation

* Counting meditation (e.g. 4–7–8 breathing, box breathing)

* Candle gazing – flame-focused meditation

Generative (meditation that evokes emotions and feelings)

This form of meditation is a mindful practice that cultivates and evokes specific emotions and feelings such as love, kindness, gratitude, forgiveness or compassion. Through intentional focus, breathwork and visualisation, this type of meditation aims to generate positive and uplifting states of being within oneself, fostering a sense of inner peace, connection and emotional wellbeing. By harnessing the power of the mind and the wisdom of the heart, generative meditation encourages the cultivation of positive qualities and fosters a deeper sense of empathy, joy and interconnectedness with ourselves and the world around us. Examples include:

* Guided meditations.

* Loving kindness meditation (heart-focused or metta meditation), which involves cultivating feelings of love, compassion and goodwill towards oneself and others through the repetition of loving phrases such as 'May you be well. May you be happy. May you be free from suffering. May you know peace.'

* Visualisation meditation or guided imagery meditation.

* Chakra meditations, which activate feelings of freedom and healing through cleansing your energy centres.

* Surrender/letting-go meditations, which involve releasing attachments, negative emotions and mental clutter by visualising and surrendering them to a higher power or the universal source.

* Gratitude meditation, which focuses on feelings of appreciation, thankfulness and abundance by reflecting on and giving thanks for various aspects of your life.

* Forgiveness meditation, where you release resentment, anger and grudges towards yourself or others by acknowledging and letting go of past hurts, mistakes and grievances.

* Inner child meditations, which involves connecting with and nurturing the inner child, healing emotional wounds and rediscovering feelings of innocence, joy and playfulness.

Awareness (self-enquiry meditation)

These are also known as contemplative, reflective or open-mind meditations. In this meditative state, you drop into a contemplative space, which involves focusing on exploring the inner self, thoughts, beliefs and emotions. I like to call these meditations **'detective of the soul meditations'**, as you ask certain questions to gain a deeper understanding of your true nature and your soul's callings. This helps to identify and release limiting beliefs or patterns. It is wonderful for taking you out of the head and into the heart.

I love using this style in my guided meditations. I bring people into the heart space, get them to breathe, release stress and then visualise the heart opening. Into this tender space I then drop a question, for example *What is my soul calling me to do?* This meditation dials down the noise of the ego and allows the voice of the soul to be heard through the emotions of the heart. Other probing questions might include: *What is it I need to know today?* or *If I truly honoured and loved myself, what would I start doing and what would I stop doing?*

This is a super meditation when you are trying to make decisions, gain clarity or simply come home to your heart.

2. Informal

These are the day-to-day ways we can weave mindfulness and meditative moments into our lives.

Mindfulness meditation

This is often known as 'present-moment awareness meditation'. It's not always easy to set aside 15–20 minutes to sit in meditation, so mindfulness meditation allows us to come back to the present moment during daily activities. Our day will often get derailed by stress, busyness or challenging situations. The act of mindfulness meditation can bring you back to a meditative state without having to sit still or be in silence. To do this:

* Stop in the middle of whatever is going on in your day.

* Close your eyes if you are able to. If not, just lower your gaze.

* Take five slow, deep belly breaths and bring your aware-ness into the body, into the heart, away from the head.

* Anchor your feet on the ground, drop your shoulders away from your ears, lengthen and strenghten your spine in order to help you find your backbone, to give you courage to face whatever challenges may be present, yet be gracious and soft through the front of your body, across the heart and chest, allowing you to have compassion, empathy and forgiveness for what is going on.

* Keep breathing deeply in and out for a few minutes until you feel your stress begin to dissipate and your body begin to feel more at ease.

When you return to your day, you will feel more anchored and aligned with a new perspective. The external stimuli might still be there, but you will react and respond differently. You will be less triggered.

If you find yourself in a situation where you are triggered or are facing a challenge, either at home or at work, you can also try the following:

* Gently excuse yourself from the room, go to the bathroom or another private space, and take some slow, deep belly breaths.

* Re-centre yourself, realign yourself, gather yourself. Place both hands on your heart and feel the connection to yourself. Feel your heart beating and say thank you for the life-force energy that is coursing through your body. Choose to use this energy for the good of yourself and others, and avoid propelling this energy into anger or rage. Continue to drop into the body. Anchor your feet by imagining them as roots attaching you solidly to the earth.

When you return to your day, you will feel more aligned, grounded and refocused.

Movement meditation (mindful movement)

Meditation doesn't have to be static. Mindful movement meditation is another powerful way to get you into flow state. This takes the form of practices that include breathwork as their anchor such as yoga, qigong, tai chi or any form of movement that really uses the breath as the gateway and focus to get out of the sympathetic side of the nervous system and into the parasympathetic side.

Other super ways include going for a mindful walk and getting out in nature. Nature therapy is a beautiful way to synchronise yourself with the rhythms of the natural world, allowing you to dial down the stress and strain of everyday burdens and life and bring you into a meditative state of coherence and harmony.

Everyday meditations

* Walking meditation: Slow down the pace at which you move from one space to the next. Tune into your bodily sensations and anchor yourself regularly to ground and come home.

* Meditate while doing your chores: Focus on your breath, play some soothing music and come into the present moment while washing the dishes, showering or cooking the dinner.

* Practise deep breathing while standing in a queue.

* Mindful eating: Savour a cup of tea without distractions, tune into the taste and texture of your food, slow your pace down, breathe between bites.

How to make meditation a daily practice

Like everything else, meditation needs practice. Just as you might do a couch to 5k programme when you start running, you will have to exercise your meditation muscle to build up your skills. But with gracious practice, it does get easier: your mind will long for it and your soul will crave it. So remember to:

* **Be patient:** It might take a while for you to be able to sit still for 10 or 15 minutes, but it will definitely be worth the effort.

* **Be consistent:** Consistency is more important than the duration of your meditation; three to five minutes every day is better than 30 minutes every second week.

* **Make it a priority:** Set time aside in your diary to do it, just as you would a meeting.

* **Create your sanctuary:** Light a candle, burn essential oils, play some relaxing music. Create your own mini spa experience. The more inviting your space, the more likely you are to go there.

* **Make it manageable:** Build mindful moments into things you are already doing, such as washing the dishes or doing the laundry.

Meditation has changed my life for the better. It's where I go to anchor and hold myself. It's my go-to place when I need to find space, seek clarity, unearth my deepest truths and listen to my soul's callings. I hope it can be that place for you too. Remember, take your time – start small and in a space where you feel safe, then let the journey inward take you home to greater mental clarity and a place of peace.

3. Mirror work – harmonising relationship to self

I believe mirror work is a powerful transformative tool, a sacred practice, and a gateway to harnessing self-love. Mirror work sets in place a positive way of thinking that eventually overrides the negative chit-chat that can inhabit your mind. It is an incredible tool for building mental fitness.

Mirror work makes us confront our innermost fears, insecurities and vulnerabilities. It gifts us the permission to embrace ourselves fully, flaws and all. It requires us to break free from self-doubt and self-criticism, enabling us to connect to our inner light, unleash our inner strength and embrace our unique beauty. As we practise mirror work regularly, we begin to see ourselves with more compassion and acknowledge ourselves for who we are.

How to practise mirror work

You can practise mirror work at any time, but doing it first thing in the morning is a great way to set yourself up for a positive day ahead.

* When you wake up, go to your mirror, plant your feet firmly on the ground, close your eyes and take a slow, deep breath. Notice any structural strains: are your shoulders tight, is your jaw clenched? Roll your shoulders down and away from your ears, stand firm, stand tall. Have a long, straight spine, strong in your back yet soft,

gracious and gentle in your front. Let your chest and heart be relaxed. Just breathe for a moment or two.

* Open your eyes and turn your gaze towards your reflection. Make gentle, gracious eye contact with yourself.

* Take a few more deep breaths to calm your mind and body, and repeat to yourself, *I am safe.*

* Begin to say some positive affirmations out loud or in your head: *I am enough, I am willing to care for myself, I am deserving of love and peace, I am loved and lovable, I am a loyal friend, a loving daughter, a caring mother* – any affirmations that resonate with you. This might be very challenging at the start, but please go gently and bear with it. You might meet resistance – negative thoughts that tell you this is crap, this is wrong, this is untrue, this is futile. All of this resistance is normal in the beginning. But if you continue with this practice, your life will be forever changed.

* Look directly into your eyes as you repeat these affirmations, feeling the words sinking in, and over time you will begin to believe them to be true. Spend at least two minutes practising mirror work to build a more loving and harmonious relationship with yourself.

* Take note of any thoughts or emotions that come up during this practice and try to respond to them with compassion and understanding and without judgement.

The kickback

Being alone with your own thoughts can be daunting, especially if you are already struggling. Saying *I am worthy* or

I am lovable can be triggering if you have just been dumped by your partner or lost your job. It can feel fake, wrong and deceitful. But if you stick with it, you will break through old limiting stories and beliefs. It exposes your pain points and reveals your shadow by evoking questions such as:

* Am I stuck in victim mode?

* Am I projecting?

* Am I repeating this same pattern again?

* Am I really that hard on myself?

* Why can I not say 'I love myself'?

* Why do I feel so much shame around my body?

* Why do I hate myself?

These might seem like drastic statements, but unfortunately this is the reality of what many people are feeling. I was shocked by the number of women who tell me they cannot look at themselves in the mirror, with some saying they have not looked at themselves in the mirror in years. The level of self-hatred and loathing is devastating. We only have one lap around this life (in this body!), so it is such a pity to see so many people in an unloving, toxic relationship with themselves. Imagine if you were married to someone who constantly told you you're ugly, fat or useless. Imagine that when you spoke, they immediately shut you up and said things like *How dare you say or think that?* or *You're so stupid.* The reality is that **you are in relationship with yourself**, and the way you speak to yourself is either creating a harmonious relationship or a toxic one that is heading to divorce. Please be kind and gentle to yourself. **The portal of pain is often the beginning of the journey home to love.** I believe the sacred ritual of daily mirror work paves the way.

4. Visualisation: design your destiny

Visualisation involves creating mental images to simulate real-life scenarios or desired outcomes. It is a powerful way of retraining your brain, as it taps into neuroplasticity, which is the brain's ability to change its function and build new neural pathways (the connections between neurons in the brain that allow for communication and information processing) that are directly related to what you are thinking about.

Take, for example, learning to play the piano. The mental skills you learn are neurological pathways. As you play the piano, you build those amazing neurological pathways in the brain, but the amazing thing is that we can build those pathways in the brain *without* playing the piano physically. If we truly visualise ourselves playing the piano, if we see our fingers and we can feel ourselves playing the piano, the brain doesn't know whether we are playing the piano for real or not, so it builds the same pathways.

Most of us are doing visualisation every single day without realising it. The danger is that we're visualising what we *don't* want, for example bad traffic, being late or a negative outcome. And so we are building the pathways, the thinking habits and the brain activity that's going to lead us to what we *don't* want instead of focusing on what we *do* want.

Visualisation also feeds the reticular activating system (RAS) of the brain. The RAS is the part of the brain related to attention and awareness. Just like a social media algorithm, whatever we express an interest in, whatever we click, whatever we like, we get more and more similar content in our feed; what we don't click, what we are not interested in, gets deleted from our feed. It is the same for the RAS: the things we think about, the conversations we have, the things we visualise all tell the brain that we are interested in those things. So the conscious brain will go into the world and find only the cues that match the story that's running in our mind, and we become blind to everything we're not thinking about.

So, every morning, visualise who you want to be. Visualise the outcome you *want*. Visualise yourself walking with confidence, speaking with courage and strength, and living with kindness. Visualise yourself falling in love or buying your dream home. This is how we fire new neurological pathways; it is how we build our new subconscious programs.

As my husband Gerry Hussey says, 'Your life cannot be any better or different than your subconscious programs. Just like a building cannot stand outside the size of its foundations, your life cannot be bigger or better or different than the size of your subconscious beliefs.'

Visualisation, when done correctly, helps you search for what you want, not what you fear.

So let's get visualising. Who is the person you want to be? What kind of life do you want to manifest? Let's flood that internal feed with images, words and stories that inspire, empower and uplift us.

Simple practices for visualisation

An audio recording in which I guide you through this meditation can be found at www.soulspace.ie/lightup with the password LIGHTUP.

Here's an easy how-to.

* Find a quiet and comfortable space, ideally where you will not be distracted. Perhaps lying in bed before getting up in the morning or at night before closing down your day.

* Close your eyes and take a few deep breaths to calm your mind and regulate your nervous system.

* Focus on a specific image, goal, situation or desired outcome. This can be anything from relaxing on a beach to a successful work event to meeting the love of your life. Imagine the details of your visualisation as clearly and vividly as possible. Use all your senses to create a picture in your mind.

* *This next part is crucial to manifesting your visualisation.* You must feel and truly embody the elevated emotions associated with your visualisation. You must go beyond just *seeing* the vision in your mind to actually embodying the emotions that are stimulated as a result of this image or goal. When you draw this image down from your head and into your heart, you flood your body with oxytocin, serotonin and dopamine – all the feel-good hormones that elevate your emotional state and raise your vibrational frequency. This then sends a signal out to the universe that you are radiating at this vibration, and **it is only when you radiate at a certain vibration that you can draw into your life whatever it is that you are trying to manifest**. Imagine that you already have what you are visualising, imagine that you are already living in that house, driving that car, in that relationship, feeling fully healthy, so that it can be attracted into your life and into your energy field.

* Stay with this visualisation for a few moments to fully immerse yourself in the experience.

∗ When you are ready, open your eyes and return to the present moment, carrying this positive motivation or energy with you. Place your hands on your heart and bow your head towards your heart in gratitude. Say a prayer or take a deep breath to close out this practice. Send out in your exhalation your desired intention, letting it float out into your energy field so that you can walk into this energy and make it manifest in your life.

Questions to visualise or to journal on

By using powerful questions, you can delve deep into your subconscious mind, uncover hidden beliefs and desires, and unlock creative potential. These prompts will encourage you to explore your inner world, set goals and manifest your dreams:

∗ Imagine yourself waking up each morning feeling energised and excited for the day ahead. How does this positive mindset shape your day and interactions with others?

∗ Visualise yourself achieving your biggest goal or dream. How does this success impact your life, relationships and overall sense of fulfilment?

∗ Envision yourself facing your biggest fear head-on and overcoming it with courage and resilience. How does this newfound sense of empowerment change your outlook on life and future challenges?

∗ Visualise the energy you want to live in and cast out every day. What type of person do you want to be? For example, the calm woman, the strong man, the grounded mother, the fearless adventurer ... Visualise how this person would show up daily, what choices they would make and the habits they have to make this future self a reality. Now go ahead and visualise yourself living this life.

Miriam's daily visualisation practice

In the morning, before I get out of bed, I love to give myself a few minutes (sometimes it only takes a minute) to visualise my day. I place my hands on my heart, close my eyes and visualise how I'd like to see myself living this day. I affirm that today is a new day, one I've never lived before, one that is filled with infinite possibilities and opportunities, and then I visualise the person I want to be that day.

Even in this short time, you can go into detail. Visualise how see yourself conversing and communicating with people, visualise your energy, how you walk, what clothes you are wearing, what you eat, how you eat, what you drink. Visualise yourself being calm, grounded, centred. Visualise yourself moving, exercising, resting. See yourself smiling, laughing, having fun ... whatever way you want your day to go. It's a very simple but effective tool for manifestation and building mental fitness.

5. Breaking through limited beliefs and habits and shifting out of subconscious programs

Through my work with clients and my own healing work, I've seen the impact and transformation that happens when we really get to the root of our core belief systems. Our thoughts, emotions and behaviours are often shaped and developed by inherited beliefs and environmental conditioning. If we truly want to change in any way, we have to be willing to do the internal excavation to break through our limiting beliefs; it is these conditioned ways of thinking that can keep us stuck, blocked and locked in life, inhibiting us from following our dreams and living up to our highest potential.

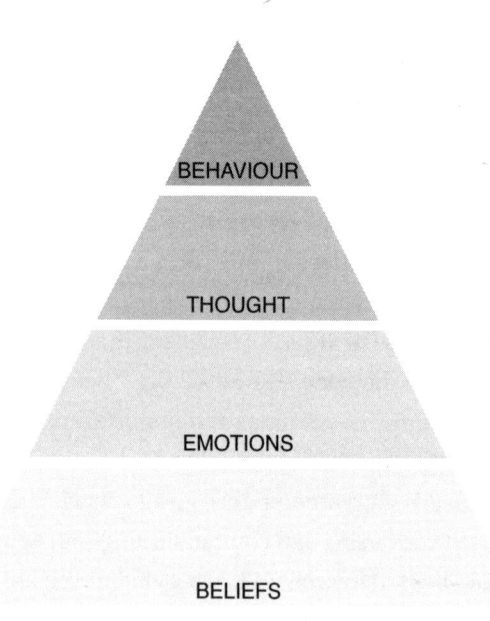

Diagram from *I Am, I Can, I Will* by Gerry Hussey

My clients often cite their behaviour as being 'the issue', for example weight gain, self-sabotaging behaviours like addictions, health concerns, relationship issues, etc. However, the behaviour is just the external symptom of a deeper issue. Unless you get to the root cause of the issue, you will never fully heal the person or their pain. Nestled underneath the behaviour is the person's thought patterns, beneath the thoughts lies their emotions, and beneath their emotional landscape rests their underlying beliefs and core values. It is our beliefs that drive our emotions, it is our emotions that drive our thinking, and it is our thinking that produces our behaviour. The behaviours then create the lifestyle.

So in order to address your lifestyle and look at lifestyle as your medicine, you must first dive beneath all the layers to unearth the roots, i.e. the belief system that each human being possesses.

What do you believe to be true about yourself? What do you believe to be true about the world? These are two powerful questions that shape the reality of your life. If you want to know what your subconscious beliefs are, you must reflect over your life (in particular, the early formative years between ages zero and seven).

The sponge effect

Ask yourself the following questions:

* What was the environment you grew up in like? Was it calm and loving or was it hostile and unsafe?

* What did you pick up along the way? What belief systems did you download? What are your conditioned beliefs?

* Who and what was celebrated in your home? Who or what was frowned upon?

* What was perceived as good and what was seen as wrong or shameful?

* What words were allowed to be said? What stories were allowed to be spoken about?

* What foods and beverages were eaten and drunk in your home?

* What roles and responsibilities did you inherit? For example, if your father went out to work long hours and worked ferociously hard, was this seen as successful? Did you subsequently inherit this core belief that to be successful you have to work really hard?

* Did you grow up in a lack-limitation household where there was poverty and scarcity? Do you now as an adult find it hard to save and be abundant? Did you download the program that there is never enough?

* Perhaps you witnessed your parents constantly rushing, running and racing. Perhaps you were never allowed to have a lie-in as that was perceived as lazy, so subsequently you downloaded the program that in order to be successful and worthy you had to be busy, you had to be productive. You earned love through what you did rather than from who you were.

As children we're constantly downloading programs, we're absorbing the energy in our environments and we're picking up on everything. I call this the sponge effect. In order to overcome self-limiting beliefs, we have to cease the conditioned beliefs. To do that, we must first become aware of what our subconscious programs are, and from there we can begin to dissect them and dilute them.

Transcending the physical and going deeper into the layers of our subconscious to extract self-limiting beliefs is imperative to healing. We must move through and transmute these imprinted programs in order to expel the myths that don't align with our deepest desires. We absorbed these beliefs from our society, our primitive and primal tribe (i.e. our family), our environment, schools and wherever we spent our early formative years (from birth to seven years). We must unstick these false 'truths' so that we can create a blank canvas on which we can imprint our own visions, truths and new beliefs that will launch us into our next chapter, creating the life that we desire and deserve from *this* moment on. I believe it's also important not to judge or criticise that which you have inherited, even if you perceive it to be bad or wrong. Your parents, teachers, caregivers and so on were doing what they knew best, given their situations and circumstances and what they had been handed down in their lifetime. Holding onto anger or hatred is futile. In order to shift out of subconscious beliefs we must do so with love and forgiveness.

In order to heal, thrive and be fully alive, we must transcend the false imprinted programs of our subconscious mind, through to the gateway of the heart and into the calling of our soul.

Breaking patterns and shifting subconscious behaviours

HABIT

We know that breaking past old programming and subconscious behaviours can be challenging, but until we learn to unblock and navigate through them, our lives will never change. For change to happen, we must be willing to investigate, challenge and shift patterns to create new beginnings and opportunities. To do this, we will use my HABIT method.

H – honesty

The key to any change in subconscious programs involves honesty with yourself. You must strip everything back to see everything within you, flaws and all, with a healthy level of curiosity and compassion for your journey, rather than judgement, shame or blame. Remember, the habits you have developed are essentially coping mechanisms to keep you safe. However, many of these habits are no longer helpful, and they can actually be harmful.

A – awareness

Before you can break old patterns, you must first become aware of the habits you want to break. Here are some ways to help you identify these habits:

* Ask friends or family for their honest feedback and opinions about your behaviours, your energy, your daily habits, your lifestyle and what they see and observe in you.

* Meditation and journalling can enable you to get clarity on your ways of being and living.

* Write out your strengths and weaknesses.

* Complete the mind, body, soul questionnaire in this book (page 14). This will highlight the areas in your life where you might be struggling. These points of strain are key indicators of where you are carrying blockages in your subconscious beliefs.

B – brainstorm

This step involves planning, organisation and visualisation. Having a map, a target or a vision is key to resetting habits and patterns. Focus on what new habits you would like to form and what old ones you'd like to replace. Here are a couple of examples of what that might look like:

Old habit Emotion Root cause	New habit (healing habit)	Plan (action)
Old habit: biting nails Emotion: anxiety, worry, fear Root cause: feeling insecure, unworthy, not enough	Finger-tracing mindfulness exercise: Hold one hand out in front of you with the fingers spread apart. Place the index finger of your other hand at the base of your thumb and begin tracing up and down the fingers. As you trace upwards, breathe in, and as you trace downwards, breathe out, giving you a total of five deep, soothing breaths. Healing habit: reduce stress and worry – use mindfulness.	Every time I go to bite my nails, I will instead be reminded to do this new exercise, send love to my hands and breathe knowing that I matter and that I am worthy.
Old habit: negative self-talk Emotion: fear, self-doubt Root cause: feeling unlovable or unloved	Say in my mind and out loud (where possible) positive affirmations about myself. Healing habit: compassion and self-care.	Every time I say something unkind or unloving to myself, I will lean into compassion and replace the unkind, unloving thought with a positive and life-affirming thought.

I – inhabit this new self

Unfortunately, 90–95 per cent of the time we are operating from subconscious programs and only 5–10 per cent of the time from our conscious mind. So, to start feeding our mind *what we do want* and *who we do want to become*, we need to fake it until we make it. Tell your mind you are already that person or have the life you dream of by acting in that way. As we learned in the visualisation section, your subconscious mind doesn't know the difference between real and imaginary, so it will play back your new programs in real life. So *get acting*!

T – track and acknowledge
The more you can track and become conscious of your changes, even if they are very subtle changes, the more sustainable, maintainable and long-lasting they will be. Acknowledging your achievements brings greater confidence. This will give you the courage to keep breaking through those limiting beliefs and keep going.

Rewiring your subconscious mind
Here are four exercises to rewire your subconscious programs. They might push you outside your comfort zone, but unless we think and act differently, nothing will change in our lives.

Write it out
Write down three to five positive mission statements that you want to become. For example, I am strong, I am confident, I am brave, I am abundant, I am beautiful.

Write out each mission statement five times every morning and evening, or as often as you can throughout the day. When we write out statements, certain areas of the brain (for example, the prefrontal cortex) light up, enabling greater processing and integration of the words. Our body 'downloads and instals' these declarations, just like a computer.

Speak out loud

Once you have made your mission statements, the next step is to speak them into existence. Saying positive mission statements out loud can activate the reticular activating system (RAS) in the brain, which we mentioned earlier. Consistently vocalising these mission statements tells your brain to focus on and seek out evidence that supports these positive beliefs. This can lead to a self-fulfilling prophecy: your beliefs shape your perceptions, emotions and actions, ultimately influencing your reality.

Say it with intent

When we write it and speak it, we *must* say it with intent – with meaning, with conviction, with passion and an unshakeable belief. We must say these affirmations from our heart, not our head. **When we say it from the heart, we flood the body with emotions – love, compassion, joy, forgiveness, peace and exhilaration**. When your body feels these emotions as though you are an embodiment of your mission statements, the subconscious mind repeats what you tell it and what it feels. So, the more the body feels these elevated emotions, the more the mind believes them to be true, and thus we rewire the brain.

Do different

Now we must do different. Nothing ever changes until *we* change. You must now start to *do* things that align to these mission statements. If your mission statement is to be fit and healthy, you must start exercising, eating healthily and engaging in lifestyle practices that will enable you to be what your mission statement says. You must go past your comfort zone, send that email, make that call, join that class. **If you want to be different, you must do different.**

Simple practices to rewire our subconscious programs

Journalling and reflection

Consider the following journalling prompts:

* What limiting beliefs about yourself are holding you back from reaching your full potential?

* What negative thoughts or self-talk do you engage in regularly, and how can you replace them with more positive affirmations?

* What childhood experiences or traumas have shaped your current beliefs about yourself and the world?

* What are some recurring patterns or behaviours in your life that you would like to change?

* How can you reframe past failures or setbacks as valuable learning experiences?

* What are some new empowering beliefs that you would like to adopt and integrate into your daily life?

* How can you practise self-love and self-compassion on a consistent basis?

* What daily practices or rituals can you implement to reinforce your new subconscious programs and create lasting change?

Meditative breathwork

An audio recording in which I guide you through this meditation can be found at www.soulspace.ie/lightup with the password LIGHTUP.

To make the shift from being led by your head to being led by your heart, try the heart-opening breath:

* Sit comfortably with your spine straight. Close your eyes. Take a few deep breaths to centre yourself and bring your awareness to your heart space.

* Begin by taking slow, deep breaths into your heart, feeling your chest expand as you inhale and relax as you exhale. Imagine breathing in love, compassion and warmth with each inhale, and releasing any tension, fear or negativity with each exhale.

* As you continue to breathe deeply into your heart, visualise your heart centre opening and expanding, radiating warmth and light throughout your entire body. Allow yourself to let go of any thoughts or worries in your mind and simply focus on the sensations in your heart space.

* You can add a mantra or affirmation to this practice, such as 'I am open to giving and receiving love' or 'I trust in the wisdom of my heart'. You can also visualise the colour green circling around your heart, or the heart as a lotus flower, opening up and expanding with each inhale. This helps to open and cleanse the heart chakra.

* Continue to breathe deeply, awakening into your heart space, for about 5–10 minutes, or as long as feels comfortable for you. Do this heart-opening breath practice daily

to cultivate a deeper connection to your heart's wisdom and your soul's whispers.

6. Self-talk: re-scripting our inner dialogue, reconstructing the narrative within and the art of reframing

Every day you tell yourself a certain story. You are either communicating it to others, or you're internally sharing messages and stories to every cell in your body through your internal narratives. Our self-talk and the stories we tell ourselves play a huge role in shaping our perception of reality, impacting our thoughts, our actions and ultimately our lives.

The most incredible lightbulb moments in my life often came as a result of expanding my awareness of the words and stories I was playing inside my head. Are you aware of the words you use to describe yourself? Some negative examples are: *Ah, that's just the way I am, I'm the clumsy one in this house, I'm the people-pleaser, I'm the peacekeeper, I'm not a runner, I'm terrible in the kitchen, I just can't lose weight, I never get a lucky break, I can never do anything right.*

Are you aware of how you describe your world? Do you see the world as a loving place filled with humanity and kindness, or do you see it as a dark, destructive space? For example, *Life is cruel, It's a hard life, We live in a dangerous world where everyone is out to get you.*

Do you speak in a positive, optimistic, loving way or is the language you use laced with pessimism, negativity, fear and jealousy? **I know everything in life is transient; however, within each of us flows a natural tendency that's associated with either the language of love and gratitude or the script of fear and negativity. This undercurrent influences the words we use, the stories we engage in and the behaviours we display.**

Would you speak to a loved one in the same way you speak to yourself? Why is it okay for us to say truly horrific things to ourselves, yet we'd never say them to someone we love? If your daughter was upset about something that happened in school, would you say, 'Ah, just shut up, forget about it, don't be such a sissy, it's probably all your fault anyway'? Would you ram wine or junk food down her throat to try to soothe and suppress it all? I'm guessing the answer is no! So why are we so hard on ourselves when we would never treat a loved one like that?

Sleep-walking through life: the wake-up call

As we now know, a lot of what we speak about can result from intergenerational programs that have been passed down to us from our ancestors. We don't just pass down eye colour and nose shape – we also pass down emotions. But we do have a choice to change these scripts. We can choose what to think, what to lean into, what we give our energy to and whether we express the language of our soul or not. The language of our soul and the language of our mind are very different. Yes, we can be bilingual and learn to speak both, but *which one* you choose to speak more of is what will manifest in your world.

The reality release: it's not all fake positivity and good vibes

If you have been hit by a storm in your life, perhaps a health crisis, the loss of a loved one, or you're living in an unsafe environment, of course you have the right to have fearful or anxious thoughts. For someone to tell you not to feel that way is wrong, for we must feel every emotion before we can move forward to heal and repair.

Transforming our inner narratives doesn't mean we ignore the struggles or pretend life is perfect. Quite the opposite. We express the struggle by speaking it out, crying it out, moving it out, breathing it out. We acknowledge these vulnerabilities and fears, and we choose to respond to ourselves with deep compassion, kindness and understanding. We must process and then release the fears and emotions, so that we can reset and begin again. From this compassionate place we can then choose to speak new stories into existence and use language that is going to enable us to keep growing towards the light.

Simple practices to change your self-talk

Reframing: transforming perspectives

Reframing has been a gamechanger in my life, particularly during stressful times and in the early years of motherhood when I was flung into the fog of it all! Instead of only seeing grey clouds I was able to see the sun peeking through. Reframing is the art of rearranging or restructuring the stories you tell to yield a different perspective on a scenario.

As you know, all words carry a certain frequency and energy, so the words you use of course impact the energy flow within your body. The word 'busy' was my nemesis. It automatically threw me into a fight or flight state and revved up my stress levels. The minute I said the word 'busy', I would feel my body tightening, my stomach would churn, and I'd feel anxious. So, I removed the word 'busy' from my life. The result? *Life-changing!* I learned to replace the word 'busy' with 'active' or 'productive' to see things from a different, more positive point of view. 'This week is an active week' is going to make you feel better mentally than 'This week is a busy week.'

We are all different, so find whatever works for you. Scan your vocabulary and when you say certain words, stop, pause and just feel into your body. Your body will tell you exactly how it feels in response to certain words. If the word causes you anxiety you might find that your stomach tightens, your shoulders drive up towards your ears, or you recoil inwards. If the word feels good to you, your stomach will soften, you might feel your shoulders drop, you might give a sigh of relief. **Upgrade your vocabulary to a language that gives you an empowering point of view and serves your soul.**

How to reframe

'I have to go to work' can be reframed as 'I get to go to work.'

'I'm blessed to have a job'; 'I get to be of service and contribute my skills and knowledge to the world.'

'I made a mistake' can be reframed as 'I have an opportunity to learn and grow from this experience.'

'I'm stuck in traffic' can be reframed as 'I have some extra time to listen to music or a podcast.'

'I'm tired' can be reframed as 'My body is telling me to rest and recharge.'

Journalling and reflection

Pay attention to the language and tone you use when you are talking to yourself. What are the first thoughts that cross your mind in the morning?

* Are they negative and self-defeating? Or are they positive and life-giving?

* Who speaks louder, your inner critic or your inner coach?

* Do you engage in a victim mentality?

* Do you engage in a lack and limitation mentality?

* Do you always find a problem or do you look for a solution?

* Do you seek out joy and compassion and celebrate yourself and your life?

* Ask yourself if there is any evidence to back up this story. Or are you just berating yourself as a result of self-defeating subconscious programs that have come to light as a result of being triggered in some way? In other words, fact check the story in your head.

Of course, we can do all these things, but which one is most dominant for you?

On reflection, are these stories serving you and helping you become the best version of yourself or are they keeping you stuck?

Cancel, clear, delete

* **Recognise the negative thought:** When you notice a negative self-talk pattern or belief arising in your mind, pause and acknowledge it without judgement. Awareness is the first step towards transformation.

* **Cancel the thought:** Mentally declare 'Cancel' or visualise pressing a Cancel button to interrupt the negative thought pattern. This action symbolises your intention to stop the thought in its tracks.

* **Clear the thought:** Next, say 'Clear' or imagine clearing out the negative thought, like deleting a file from your mental space. Visualise a white light or a sweeping motion that cleanses and purifies your mind from the negative energy.

* **Delete the thought:** Finally, say 'Delete' or envision pressing a Delete button to permanently erase the negative thought from your mental landscape. Focus on releasing the thought with love and compassion.

* **Replace with a positive affirmation:** After cancelling, clearing and deleting the negative thought, introduce a positive affirmation or mantra to replace it.

Seek support

Opening up to trusted friends, family members or mental health professionals about negative self-talk can provide validation and perspective. Talking through our thoughts and feelings with others can help us gain insight and develop healthier coping strategies.

The stories we tell ourselves, the thoughts we think and the pictures we create in our minds are the biggest dictators of the life we lead. Choose your words carefully. Consciously say something nice to yourself or a loved one first thing in the morning. Remember, energy flows where your thoughts go. Changing your story will change your day. Changing your days will change your life.

7. Affirmations: uplifting declarations for life

An affirmation is a statement that we say to ourselves (either in our mind or out loud to the world). We often hear of 'positive affirmations', which we will explore; however, it is imperative to understand that you are affirming things to yourself every day whether or not you know it. As discussed earlier, many of these things are generated from your subconscious mind, as we are running on autopilot most of the time.

They might be positive affirmations or they might be negative. Now that you are fully aware that you are constantly affirming things in your mind, it is empowering to know that you have a transformative potion: positive affirmations.

Positive affirmations are statements that you *consciously* choose to repeat regularly, either by saying them or writing them. The more you repeat the affirmation the more it lodges in your mind, the more it takes up residency and space, and, almost like osmosis, these positive statements begin to sink into your subconscious mind and become real.

As the beautiful quote from the Buddha goes:

> *Our life is shaped by our mind; we become what we think. Suffering follows an evil thought as the wheels of a cart follow the oxen that draws it. Our life is shaped by our mind; we become what we think. Joy follows a pure thought like a shadow that never leaves.*
> *Buddha*

How to use affirmations

Do:

* Create your own personal affirmations. It is much more impactful when you make affirmations your own. Use ones that really open your heart and that ring true for you.

* Repeat your affirmations daily, ideally in the morning or at night before bed. Consistency is key in making them a habit.

* Say them out loud, couple them with looking in the mirror, gazing into your precious eyes. (This will supercharge your affirmations, making you manifest them even faster.)

* Say your affirmations with conviction. This will reinforce the positive beliefs in your mind.

* Visualise yourself already embodying these affirmations. Feel these emotions and sensations flow through your body, opening your heart and elevating your vibration.

Don't:

* Choose negative affirmations. Affirmations should always be laced with enthusiasm and be framed in a positive light.

* Rely solely on affirmations to change your life. We must put the work in in all areas of our life. Scaffolding affirmations onto other lifestyle changes is key.

* Give up. It takes time for affirmations to make a long-lasting impact. It takes time for the subconscious program to be rewired.

* Get derailed by imposter syndrome or feeling like you're not enough. If the affirmation feels fake to you initially, keep affirming it anyway – it is only by repetition that you get to create your new script.

If you are struggling to come up with your own affirmations, here are some ideas to get you going.

Affirmations for prosperity and abundance

* I attract wealth and abundance with gratitude and ease. I am a magnet for abundance in all areas of my life.

* The universe provides me with endless opportunities to prosper and succeed. I say Yes to life.

* I am worthy of all the prosperity and abundance that comes my way.

* I now step into the winning circle of my life. Money flows to me in unexpected and miraculous ways.

* I release all limiting beliefs about money and open myself up to receive unlimited abundance.

* I deserve to live a life of prosperity and abundance, and I allow it to flow into my life effortlessly.

Affirmations for stepping outside your comfort zone

* I release all fear and doubt. I am divinely protected. This protection enables me to boldly step into the realm of possibility and potential.

* On the other side of this cave of uncertainty lie my greatest opportunities for success, renewal and transformation.

* I am capable of facing new challenges and thriving in unfamiliar situations.

* I trust in my abilities to adapt and navigate through the unknown with grace and resilience.

* I am open to learning and growing through discomfort, knowing that it is a natural part of my evolution and transformation.

* I trust in my intuition to guide and support me as I navigate new horizons.

Affirmations for when you are scared

* I am safe and protected. I trust that everything is unfolding for my highest good.

* I breathe in courage and exhale fear, grounding myself in the present moment.

* Every emotion is temporary. This too shall pass.

* I am brave. I am stronger than my fears. I can do this.

* I am surrounded by love and support; I can lean on others when I feel scared. I am divinely supported and protected.

* I am a warrior of light, and I shine brightly even in the darkest moments.

Affirmations for health and healing

* I nourish my body with nutritious foods and beverages and my mind with uplifting thoughts and stories. I make choices that nourish me at a cellular level.

* Every cell in my body is healing. It is being graced by divine light and is vibrating with positive energy and vitality.

* I am grateful for the healing that is taking place within me, physically, mentally, emotionally and spiritually.

* I listen to my body. I take time to rest and recover, allowing my body to heal and recharge.

Affirmations for courage, strength and inner belief

* I am strong. I am capable. I can handle whatever comes my way today.

* An inner strength resides within me. I am a warrior of humanity. A depth of courage springs from my soul. I am competent and capable.

* I tap into the unlimited potential source energy of the universe. I am an infinite being, living in an infinite universe. I believe in my unlimited potential to achieve my dreams and goals. Anything and everything is possible. *If not me, then who?*

* Despite adversities, I know I am resilient and strong. I'm a beacon of courage, strength and self-belief, shining brightly in all that I do.

* I trust in my inner strength to guide me, protect me and raise me up.

Affirmations for forgiveness

* I release any feelings of anger or resentment. I choose to forgive and let go. I choose to let my soul free.

* I deserve peace and freedom, so I forgive and let go.

* Forgiveness is a gift I give myself. I move on with graciousness and love. I send love to all those who have wronged me, including myself. I forgive and I am free.

* Forgiveness is a powerful act of love and liberation. I choose to forgive and set myself free.

* I forgive others for their mistakes and flaws, knowing that we are all imperfect beings. I let go of the burden of hurt.

* Forgiveness is a choice, and I choose to let go of the past and move forward with peace and compassion.

Affirmations for dealing with loss and grief

* I allow myself to grieve. I give myself permission to feel and process my emotions in my own time and in my own way. I tread softly and allow myself to have reverence for this tender time.

* I acknowledge that it's okay to feel sadness and pain during this time.

* I find comfort in cherished memories and the love that still remains.

* I trust that healing is a natural process and that I will move through it in my own way and at my own pace.

* I ride the waves of grief as they come and go. When a big wave hits, I allow myself to be vulnerable. When the wave subsides, I give myself permission to feel love and cherish fond memories. I allow the light to enter and the darkness to lift.

* I go gently through this difficult process and trust that I will emerge from this chrysalis with greater strength, compassion and love.

Affirmations for anxiety and overwhelm

* I breathe in courage and exhale fear. I am safe and secure. All is well in my world.

* I am resilient and brave. I can navigate through difficult situations. From this situation only good will come. I trust everything is happening for my highest good.

* I am safe and supported by the universe and am held by Mother Earth. I feel roots grounding me to the earth, keeping me solid, safe, secure and strong. I ground down so that I can fly high.

8. Re-centring routines: calming and revitalising practices to realign focus and trigger positive transformations

Our brain takes up a lot of energy, so it needs rest to perform at its best. It can function optimally for up to 90 minutes. After this, if we don't take a break, concentration diminishes and it continues to diminish until we rest and recharge.

So, every 90 minutes, it is important to reset what we're doing. For example, set an alarm for 90 minutes when you're at your desk. When it goes off, get up, maybe take a stretch, shake things out, get a glass of water, go to the bathroom, go outside, walk around your house or office, or do some deep breathing. This helps you to realign, refocus and improve mental agility, performance and clarity. When you go back to your desk you're coming back with a renewed freshness.

Routines and rituals

Having a morning routine is an important way to wake up and greet your new day. It eliminates that morning rush, which inevitably leads to a 'grab and go' breakfast and sends out a chaotic signal to your energy field, almost like you're chasing a wild horse for the day.

The energy you wake up in, the emotions you feel and the thoughts you meet the day with have the power to dictate how your day will run. You either attack your day with vengeance or you greet your day with openness. Creating a peaceful morning ritual helps create a peaceful day, which in turn results in a more peaceful life.

Below are some useful ideas that you can try to incorporate into your own morning routine.

Mental wellbeing

* Morning affirmations

* Visualisations

* Self-talk: Change your narrative and internal stories to ones that are life-affirming, inspiring and encouraging

* Acknowledgement: Create mini win lists

* Self-compassion: Be kind, be open, be willing.

Emotional wellbeing

* Meditation, prayer, silence

* Gratitude

* Breathwork (e.g. diaphragmatic breathing, box breathing, 4–7–8 breathing, alternate nostril breathing – see pages 274–5)

* Mirror work

* Journalling.

Physical wellbeing

* Hydration and morning elixir: Warm water and lemon (with ginger if you like it) on waking, 15–30 minutes before food.

* Movement: Gentle stretching, dancing, skipping, bouncing, boxing, swimming, walking, running, cycling – anything that gets you moving!

* Nutritional fuelling: Balanced, wholesome, real-food breakfast.

* Morning light: Within 15 minutes of waking, expose yourself to sunlight (or if you wake before the sun rises, turn on the lights in your home) to help with circadian rhythms and sleep cycles.

* Lymphatic drainage techniques and mindful teeth-brushing.

Soulful wellbeing

* Connection: Hug someone or something (a pet, a teddy bear) *and* hug yourself to release oxytocin.

* Soulful music: Music can raise vibration and it's a feel-good factor. Switch off negative radio/TV.

* Environment: Ensure the environment you wake up in every day is a clear, clean, decluttered and inspiring one. A cluttered environment = a cluttered, anxious mind.

* I love you: Ensure you say the words 'I love you' to someone each morning (either in person or by text or phone call) and/or say them to yourself.

* Nature's therapy: Get outside in the fresh air to clear the mind and cleanse the soul.

Try out new rituals; use your body as a lab and find out what feels good for *you*. We are all beautifully unique, so listen to your body and honour its needs. To create healthy night-time routines see the sleep section on page 120.

Each day is one you have never, ever lived before: it has infinite possibilities and opportunities. Miracles are waiting to unfold if we just allow ourselves to see the beauty and the wonder both in ourselves and all around us. Creating daily rituals brings you into the present moment, the present day, which is all we ever have.

9. Forgiveness: the freeing power of forgiving

Forgiveness unblocks the heart and opens the channels for love to flow again.

I believe forgiveness is one of the greatest gateways to freedom, emotional health and greater happiness. Forgiveness is the ability to choose where we place our energy and attention. Forgiveness is not about condoning the past; it's not about saying that what happened or how people behaved was right or acceptable. It is about making a powerful decision that ensures we are no longer attaching our energy, attention or awareness to that thing, person or place.

Forgiveness is where we decide to release all the unhelpful emotions of anger or bitterness for the sake of our health and happiness. Forgiveness can involve forgiving ourselves, others or the universe. We all have different pasts; some of us have every right to be angry and bitter. Nobody can deny you that. But ask yourself: if you continue to hold that anger, if you continue to give away your power and freedom to that place, time or person, how does that impact the rest of your life?

First and foremost, **forgiveness is a gift to self**. It is the gateway to emotional freedom. Who or what do you need to forgive? What would it take for you to give yourself permission to forgive and be free? If you were no longer giving your time or energy to the past or to that person, and you were to now put that time and energy into something new, something exciting or something loving, what would that feel like?

We will all experience challenges in our lives when someone's behaviour is triggering and you hold a resentment or anger towards that person. This is normal, but learning to forgive can be one of the most powerful gateways to liberating your soul. When we hold a resentment towards someone we only hurt ourselves, because it lowers our energy and our vibrational frequency, and it dims our enthusiasm for life. When we look at a situation through the lens of forgiveness, we can see that a person's unkind deeds and words are usually a reflection of their own inner turmoil or pain.

When people act unkindly towards you, they eclipse the light and love from their own life. If you hold on to the resentment, hurt, anger and pain, you too eclipse light and love from your life. Forgiveness can be a challenging thing to do, especially if you feel you have been wronged or betrayed in the most unloving or unkind way. But do not be caged by the ravenous anger that can destroy your life. By staying stuck in anger, you actually give the power over to the person who has done the unkind deed. They now become victorious, they have now taken your light and love away, so to forgive does not mean that you forget, ignore or suppress, it does not mean that you now have to spend time in the company of those people who seem to have unkindly behaved towards you – you can distance yourself with love, you can keep moving forward with love, but you will never forget. From each experience, you will gain lessons and valuable insights that will contribute to your growth and evolution.

When you engage in the act of forgiveness, deep healing can occur on many levels:

* It frees you from pain, anger, hurt and anguish.

* It reduces physical pain, inflammation and illness. Studies from Johns Hopkins and Luther College have found that forgiveness has a whole range of health benefits.

* It dissolves the wavelengths, energy and frequency of anger, fear and pain from emanating from your aura or energy field. Since you attract what you think about, by cutting the cords to this negative or anger energy you begin to untangle yourself from more situations or scenarios that might manifest in your world. We want to repair, not repeat.

* Forgiving also heals the other person. Life has potentially hardened them and, believe it or not, beneath their pain is a deep longing for love.

Simple practices to forgive

Affirmations

Try practising this beautiful affirmation: 'I am willing to forgive. I am willing to set myself free. I release anger and invite peace.'

Reflective exercises

Engage in a forgiveness ritual such as lighting a candle, saying a prayer, writing a letter and burning it, or throwing a rock off the side of a mountain. These symbolic gestures signify your intention to forgive and let go. Use this ritual as a sacred space to release grievances and invite healing and reconciliation into your heart.

Journalling

Reflect on a situation in your life where you are holding on to resentment or anger towards someone. How is this emotional burden impacting your wellbeing and your relationships? What beliefs or fears may be preventing you from forgiving this person? Now consider a time when you have been forgiven by someone else. How did this act of grace and compassion make you feel? Reflect on the power of forgiveness in healing and transforming relationships.

Breathwork

Start by focusing on your breath, noticing the sensation of air entering and leaving your body. Begin to bring the person, place or thing against whom you hold a grudge into your mind's eye. Bring your awareness and breath to the heart centre and begin to connect with the pain and hurt stored in your heart. Through slow and deep breaths, allow the emotions to surface and then release them gently through the exhale. As you continue to breathe deeply and consciously into the heart, begin the process of loving kindness. To do this, begin to inhale and imagine breathing in feelings of love, compassion and kindness, and silently repeat: *May you be happy. May you be healthy. May you be free from suffering and pain. May you be safe and may you find peace.*

Continue to breathe in love and kindness and send these positive blessings to this person, place or thing. Then begin to bring yourself into your mind's eye, breathing deeply, and then drop your awareness into your heart.

As you inhale, imagine breathing in feelings of love, compassion and kindness, and silently repeat the following: *May I be happy. May I be healthy. May I be free from suffering and pain. May I be safe and may I know peace.*

By repeating this practice often, you may find that you are able to shift your perspective and begin to see the situation from a place of compassion and understanding, paving the way for forgiveness.

10. Gratitude: the graceful path to heartfelt appreciation

Gratitude is a gamechanger: it is life-transforming, heart-opening and it brings a glimmer of joy to your world even in the darkest times. Gratitude is the appreciation of what is valuable and meaningful to you, and where you intentionally focus on the good things in your life.

Gratitude is the process of giving yourself some time and space to reflect on the blessings in your life. It truly is that simple, yet it has the power to enhance our physical, mental, emotional, psychological and social sense of wellbeing.

When you intentionally focus on the good things in your life, you start to practise deeper awareness. This, in turn, enables you to live a life of more ease and grace. When you focus on the things that are good and well in your life, you start to rewire your brain to reduce negativity bias. Negativity bias is our default, which means we are more likely to focus our attention on threat. However, if we don't consciously make an effort to reverse our negativity bias, we might likely find ourselves living a very pessimistic way of life. Gratitude is a powerful antidote to pessimism, and it can spin you around into living a more optimistic life where you notice and engage in greater opportunities. When you focus on the small wins in your life, you start to rewire your brain to focus on your blessings and attract more of that into your life. This is the process of neuroplasticity (as previously mentioned), where you rewire your brain by focusing on what you want rather than what you don't want. You can now draw in more of what you're putting back out.

Gratitude really is about finding the extraordinary in the ordinary. It's paring it right back to being grateful for the simple things in your life: that warm cup of tea in the morning, the magical sunset in the evening, the melody of the birds singing in the trees, a random smile from a stranger, making eye contact with the person you love, that snuggle from your mother, a hug from a friend. The more we tune into those micro magical moments, the more we change the physiology, the chemistry, the biology of the body. We flood our body with life-giving, life-serving feelings with the release of serotonin, dopamine and oxytocin, and we deactivate stress and inflammatory markers in the body. **Gratitude can be the greatest super-pill you will ever take, and it doesn't cost anything and has zero side effects.**

Benefits of gratitude

The benefits of gratitude, as you might have guessed already, are vast. It benefits us psychologically (mentally and emotionally) physically and socially.

Psychological

* **Activation of neurotransmitters:** This leads to increased mood and feelings of wellbeing and happiness through the release of the hormones serotonin, dopamine and oxytocin.

* **Reduced depression:** According to some research studies, writing a letter of gratitude can vastly reduce feelings of hopelessness and increase levels of optimism.

* **Reduced stress:** Gratitude deactivates the amygdala area, switching off the hormones of stress, which dials down the activation of the sympathetic part of the nervous system, allowing the body to become more regulated.

* **Enhanced resilience and grit:** Practising gratitude makes you more resilient and able to withstand challenges and overcome trauma in your life.

* **Neuroplasticity:** Practising gratitude regularly builds neural pathways in the brain, developing neuroplasticity and allowing you to become more naturally optimistic and opportunistic rather than pessimistic in your life.

* **Greater internal confidence, clarity and performance:** Gratitude helps you dial down the noise, the busyness and the chaos so the storms within can subside.

Physical

* **Better sleep:** Practising gratitude can help with sleep by reducing the clutter in your mind. Engaging in gratitude before bed can be a great cleansing practice to release any negative thought patterns that might be replaying in your mind.

* **Reduced blood pressure:** Once you begin to switch off the sympathetic side of the nervous system and drop more into a balanced state of living, blood pressure will reduce.

* **Enhanced immune system:** According to a study (UC Davis Health Study 2015), the practice of gratitude contributes to reducing the biomarkers of inflammation by 7 per cent among individuals diagnosed with congestive heart failure.

Social

* **Greater empathy, relationships and social connections:** If you practise gratitude, you are likely to express and share feelings of love, respect, acknowledgement, compassion and joy. If you are a person who is innately more joyful, naturally you're going to attract and be in more loving, kind, harmonious relationships.

* **More likeable among team members:** Gratitude gives you a sense of increased self-esteem and greater internal confidence. This greater self-esteem enables you to become more engaged, more vocal, more likely to stand out, to put your hand up and become more connected, making you more favoured by team members and peers.

* **Decreased social comparisons:** People who practise gratitude are more likely to practise non-judgement and non-comparison. Gratitude is a super-powerful tool to strengthen our internal muscle of greater confidence and love. With the prevalence of social media, we need to enhance, grow and instigate greater emphasis on practising gratitude, especially imparting this wisdom to the

next generation, so that we can elevate and overcome social comparisons and feel more internal ease.

* **Enhanced pro-social behaviour:** Gratitude has a powerful way of allowing people to be of more service to the world. The serotonin and dopamine flooding through your system can enable you to be kinder, opening you up to engage in charitable and volunteer work, random acts of kindness and generally just being an overall caring person. The ripple effect of gratitude is life-serving and giving to everybody.

Simple practices to express gratitude

Gratitude jar or collage

This involves writing down things you are grateful for on small pieces of paper and putting them in a jar to read later. This simple practice can help shift your focus away from negative, fear-based thoughts towards cultivating a mindset of appreciation and abundance. At the end of the year it can be particularly beautiful and heartwarming to read all these notes and relive some of the moments of magic.

Create a gratitude collage or vision board to visually represent the things you are grateful for in your life. Use images, words and symbols that evoke feelings of thankfulness and abundance. Display your collage in a place where you can see it daily to cultivate a mindset of appreciation and positivity, for example on your fridge door, on your bedside locker, in your wallet or as a screensaver on your laptop or phone.

Express and share

Make it a daily habit to express gratitude to others by saying thank you, whether to a colleague, a family member, a friend or even a stranger who has helped you in some small way. By expressing and sharing gratitude, you send the vibration of love and appreciation into your energetic fields, enabling you to create and manifest more of that back into your life. Engaging in random acts of kindness is another great way to express gratitude.

Gratitude journalling

Simply write down each morning three things you are grateful for, no matter how big or small. This practice can help you focus on the positive aspects in your life, increase your overall sense of wellbeing and improve your mood for the day ahead. Closing down your day by also writing three things into your gratitude journal can be a wonderful way to reflect back over the day. Capturing your mini wins can boost confidence and give you a sense of appreciation before you go to sleep, carrying the energy of gratefulness with you. I'd encourage you to invest in a journal, one that feels comforting and beautiful to you. Leave it on your bedside locker as an invitation to explore your inner world and create that sanctuary of gratitude and build up that muscle of positivity.

Gratitude letter-writing

Writing a heartfelt letter to someone you love detailing how they have impacted your life positively and why you are grateful for their presence is a wonderful way to express gratitude. Consider sharing this letter with them for an added emotional connection.

Breathwork

To do gratitude breathwork, simply find a comfortable space, close your eyes or lower your gaze to the tip of your nose and turn your gaze inwards, focusing on your breath. As you inhale, let your belly, ribcage, chest and heart area expand, and think about things that make you happy and that you are truly grateful for. As you exhale, let your belly and chest fall, releasing tension, stress or strains. Place an image of something, someone or some place that you are grateful for into your heart. Focus on opening your heart by imagining a warm light surrounding your chest area. Visualise this glowing light expanding with each breath, emanating love, gratitude and grace. Repeat this practice for a few minutes to help cultivate and deepen those feelings of gratitude and appreciation.

11. Nutrition, hydration and gut health

What we consume, as we know from the section on nutritional wellbeing, is extremely important for mental fitness. Making sure that you're adequately hydrated, looking at your nutrition and minding your gut health is vital for fuelling your mind for enhanced clarity and performance.

For more information on all of this, refer back to Chapter 4.

Master the mind and master your life. A calm mind is one of the greatest catalysts to internal peace and physical ease. As we say at Soul Space, 'Change your thinking, change your world.'

Light-up moments for the mind

◊ Curling up with a new inspiring book that transports you to another world

◊ A song or smell that brings back good memories

◊ Listening to an uplifting podcast or music that liberates your mind

◊ Reading a quote that resonates and inspires with you

◊ Going for a carefree drive and listening to your favourite playlist

◊ Insightful conversations that stimulate your mind and awaken inspiration

◊ The calming sensation in your mind after meditating or being immersed in nature

◊ The clarity, relief and togetherness after dumping all your negative thoughts onto a page

◊ Reflecting and planning for the week ahead

◊ Long walks and deep chats

◊ Permission to switch off and be unproductive without the guilt

◊ Checking items off your to-do list

◊ Morning quiet time

◊ Saying affirmations that make you feel strong, confident, loved and aligned.

SOUL

We are all different. We are all made up of energy and information, but we are all sequenced together differently by the presence of our soul. Please don't judge or compare yourself against another. Be you. Embrace originality and diversity. Express what's in your heart and soul.

CHAPTER 7

SOULFUL ILLUMINATION: EMBRACING THE LIGHT WITHIN

I believe spirituality is one of the biggest pillars missing from today's model of wellness. Without spirituality, how do we know who we are? If we don't know who we are, how can we possibly live a life that is authentic? How can we become the best, most invigorated version of ourselves? How can we seek to serve the world as we are meant to, shining our unique gifts and talents, if we don't know who we are or what our purpose is? Connecting to our soul through spirituality allows us to honour the beauty and peace that lies within, so that we can connect to the greater wisdom of the universe. This is key to feeling whole and having true health and vitality. The soul makes no mistakes. We focus so much on the physical, the mental and emotional, but the missing link, I believe, is the presence and magical power of the soul in illuminating your life. **If you supercharge your soul, you supercharge your life.**

In this section, we will delve into the profound essence of the soul and unravel its interconnectedness with our health and wellbeing. We will explore the transformative tools that enable us to connect with and access our soul, allowing us to embark on a journey to unlock, expand and liberate our spiritual self. Through this journey, we will highlight the various ways we can allow our soul to shine, luminously radiate and light up.

What is your soul?

I believe your soul is your essence. It is the sacredness that resides within you. It's your energy, it's who you are at the very core of your being: your true self, your personality, your purpose, your passion, your dreams. It is the seat of your desires and consciousness. When you are conceived and enter into your mother's womb, you enter as a sparkle of light, as stardust that grows into a seed, which then becomes a physical being. When your time comes to depart this earth, the vessel or vehicle of your body disintegrates into dust, but your soul lives on. **Your soul is infinite, a never-ending spark of energy and light**. It is boundless love, purity and grace. You cannot exist without your soul. It is *you*. It is what makes you so special. Even though the soul is unseen and invisible (to most people), it is very much the heart of who you are. It holds the imprints from all your lifetimes, it holds your karma, your truths, your past experiences, creating a complex web that influences your present and shapes your future.

I believe the soul is the centre point from which everything else emanates – our 'everything' is contained within this ethereal force guiding us on our journey through life and beyond. As we navigate through the complexity of life, it is our soul that acts as our compass, guiding us towards our highest potential and ultimate purpose.

Your soul is an infinite field of energy

According to many spiritual and metaphysical beliefs, the soul is not bound by the confines of time, space or the physical body; it is a limitless source of energy that transcends the material world. **Einstein said that energy cannot be created or destroyed, it can only be changed from one form to another.** Take water, for example: it can take on many forms, such as liquid, ice or steam, but the total amount of water remains constant. When water evaporates and condenses into clouds, the energy is transferred from the water molecules to the surrounding air molecules. Eventually the water falls back to the earth as rain or snow, releasing this stored energy.

One way to understand the soul as an infinite field of energy is to consider it as a non-physical, eternal essence that contains the ember of who we are as individuals. This energy is constantly evolving and growing, with the potential for infinite expansion and transformation.

Many spiritual traditions also believe that the soul is connected with all other forms of energy in the universe, and that it has the ability to influence and interact with the world around us in profound ways. This interconnectedness is often described as a 'universal life-force energy' and it is present in all beings.

Ignition and illumination of the soul

Of course, as we've already discussed in this book, all the other pillars of wellbeing are important; however, the true foundations of solid health stem from whether or not your soul is ignited. **Our soul is our ultimate nest. It is our haven, our safe space. It's the ultimate keeper of our individual**

truths. It is the mirror of our innermost beauty, and it is the divine eternal flame that burns brightly within us – our shining light that guides us forwards and towards connection, truth and oneness with the universe. It is the home of our divine light. Just as a hot air balloon cannot take flight without the invisible gas to ignite it, our soul is the invisible force that ignites our life.

If you are living a life in alignment with your soul's calling, your light shines out brightly in all directions. When you're attuned to it, you naturally exude charisma, charm, joy, fun, ease and grace. You're the type of person who will light up the room, irrespective of what size you are or what clothes you wear. It's your energy that lights up the room, not how you look.

If you're in tune with your soul's calling, your light shines bright like a beam of sunlight, shining down upon the earth, glistening upon the ocean, shimmering across the sky, lighting up everything it touches and connects with. There's strength, power, meaning and purpose to it. It's a ray of hope, love, inspiration and beauty.

If you're not living in alignment with your soul's true calling – perhaps you're living a life that you *think* you should be living, or living a life that isn't a right fit for who you are – your light might still shine, but it will flicker faintly, resembling the artificial light of a torch rather than the illuminating light force of the sun. The light from the sun is natural, radiant and strong. A torch's light is fake, timid and doesn't have as much depth or power. Ask yourself, are you a sun beaming brightly or are you a torch flickering dimly?

The body is where our soul resides. If we have an unwell soul, we will create an unwell body. Honour the soul. Honour the body. Honour your life.

What is spirituality?

Spirituality is any ritual that connects you to your soul and deepens your connection to the oneness of the universe. Accessing your soul through spiritual self-care practices is imperative for greater wellbeing on so many levels. Spirituality has different meanings to different people, often influenced by the ideologies they grew up with. Maybe you associate spirituality with religion or cultural traditions. Perhaps you associate it with nature or the universe, or art, music or dance. Ultimately, it can be anything that is meaningful to you.

Often spirituality is misinterpreted as religion. It can be religion for many; however, it is often more than any doctrine-controlled institution. God plays a huge role in my life. Without God, I'd be lost. Prayer is my sanctuary. Church is my safe place. But spirituality, when we really break it down, is anything that gets you off the treadmill of life for a while. It allows you to drop into your inner space, which is calm, peaceful and nurturing. Spirituality is anything that allows you to tune in to the deep intuitive messages from your gut, the true callings from your heart and the whispers from your soul. Engaging in a spiritual way of living through daily spiritual practices allows you to live a life of ease and grace. A life of less stress and distraction.

What brings you alive? What ignites your soul? When and where do you feel at home, at peace, in flow state? This may be on your yoga mat, out in nature, in church or whilst meditating. Finding what brings you peace and joy is key to finding what spiritual practices best serve you.

Without spirituality we can end up being 'homeless souls'. We can create voids within ourselves that can never be filled with possessions, food, drugs, alcohol, job promotions or Instagram followers. We must fill up our soul from the inside out by truly spending time each day in silence and stillness so that we can connect to and hear the true calling of the soul. To truly become whole and embrace spirituality we must also prioritise doing things daily that we love and that light us up.

Prioritising your spirituality can:

* Improve your relationships and connections with others

* Enable you to experience more inner ease and peace

* Help you gain clarity on what makes you happy

* Enhance feelings of oneness and universality

* Diminish feelings of isolation and loneliness

* Deepen your relationship with self

* Allow joy, fun, light and love to flow

* Improve your mental, emotional and physical health and vitality.

Access to the soul: opening the gateway to your innermost self through the breath

Our breath is a gateway to meeting ourselves beyond the noise. It is the entryway to attuning to our feelings, listening to our hearts and honouring our needs. It is the gateway to healing, the portal to peace and the channel that connects us to the divine.

Access to the soul via the breath has long been a practice in various spiritual traditions. The breath serves as a gateway to our soul, a pathway that allows us to navigate past the external layers of noise and distraction, away from the physical sensations, from the mental chatter, to arrive at our true essence, which is divine grace and love.

Your breath is the first thing that enters your body when you are born and it's the last thing to leave when you die. Without breath we are nothing. Most people do not fully use the power of the breath to truly enhance their health and wellbeing, but the good news is that with patience, attention, awareness and a little coaching, anybody can learn how to engage more effectively with their breath for optimal health and vitality. While it's not a magic bullet for all life's challenges or difficulties, I believe that engaging in conscious and intentional daily breathwork can root us more deeply in our bodies and take us home to our souls.

When you engage in breathwork, you gain access to yourself in a way that is markedly different to that of your baseline waking self. You can enter into a deeper state of consciousness where you become more aware, and in this state a vast amount of unconscious information is made conscious. A lot of the things you may have been blind to can suddenly emerge, almost as if you have had a conversation with a wiser, older or future version of yourself. Going deep into breathwork can shift your perspective, allowing you to see more clearly and make life decisions that are more aligned to your innermost truths and your soul's callings.

Breathwork benefits

Our bodies are designed to clear out unnecessary material in a variety of ways, including through the breath. It is a process of detoxification in which unwanted stale energy is expelled. The exhale is a necessary component of clearing energetic, physical and emotional debris. As you begin to pay closer attention to your breath, you will learn to decipher when you are in a stressed or reactive state, allowing you then to use your breath as a tool to take action, to shift your breathing away from stress and strain, and to invite in moments of calm, clarity and healing. The breath ignites the flow of prana/chi or life-force energy, connecting the entirety of our being: from the physical (inward flow of oxygen) to the mental, emotional and spiritual.

As well as stress relief, the benefits of breathwork include:

* **Improved mental clarity and focus:** Deep-breathing exercises can increase oxygen flow to the brain, leading to improved concentration, cognitive function and mental clarity.

* **Enhanced emotional wellbeing:** Breathwork can help release emotional blockages, trauma and negative emotions stored in the body, leading to a greater sense of emotional balance, peace and overall wellbeing. (Please note: when dealing with trauma, rapid, intense breathwork practices like holotropic breathing, forced breathing or breath holding should only be practised in a safe place with trained professionals.)

* **Increased energy levels:** Deep-breathing exercises can help improve oxygen circulation in the body, leading to

increased energy levels, vitality and a greater sense of wellbeing.

* **Improved physical health:** Breathwork can have a positive impact on various aspects of physical health, such as improving lung function, boosting the immune system, reducing inflammation and lowering blood pressure.

* **Better sleep:** Relaxation and breathing exercises can help calm the mind and body, leading to improved sleep quality and better overall sleep patterns.

* **Increased self-awareness and mindfulness:** Breathwork encourages self-awareness and mindfulness by helping individuals connect with their breath, body and emotions, leading to a greater sense of presence and awareness in the present moment.

* **Deeper connection to spiritual and intuitive guidance:** It is the gateway to uncaging the soul and letting it be free.

Types of breathing to help access the soul

Breathwork is known as pranayama in yoga. It was defined by the yoga guru Patanjali as the 'regulation and control of the inhalation and exhalation of the breath, creating luminosity and preparing the mind for one-pointed focus'. A regular and sustained practice of pranayama not only amplifies our entire body but prepares our mind for deep meditation and super-charges the soul.

There are many different types of breathwork, some of which you have already encountered in this book. A few of the main ones are described below. If you have never done breathwork before, a good place to start is with deep diaphragmatic or belly breathing – it is simple yet effective, and it can be done anywhere. As you become more used to deep breathing, you can branch out and try some new forms, enabling you to untangle from external stresses and deepen into the essence of your soul.

These breathwork practices are wonderful ways to help balance the nervous system, calm the mind, reduce stress and anxiety, increase mental clarity, bring a sense of peace and centredness and gain deeper access to the soul's internal wisdom.

Diaphragmatic breathing

Of all of the breathing techniques and pranayama tools I have learned over the past 20 years, one of the most well known and transformative, I believe, is the simple act of deep belly breathing, or diaphragmatic breathing.

To practise, start by sitting or lying down in a comfortable position. Place one hand on your chest and the other hand on your abdomen. Inhale deeply through your nose, allowing your abdomen to expand and rise. Pause at the top of the inhale for a few seconds and, when you are ready, exhale slowly through your mouth or nose, letting your abdomen fall and contract. Repeat this breathing technique for several minutes, focusing on the sensation of your belly rising and falling with each breath.

Counting breathing

Counting breathwork involves the simple act of counting each breath as you breathe deeply. This technique allows you to stay focused while enabling your nervous system to relax and become more centred and grounded. To do this counting breathwork, simply sit or lie down in a quiet place. Turn your awareness inwards by closing your eyes or lowering your gaze and take deep, slow breaths. Begin counting your breaths, starting at one for each inhale and exhale. If your mind wanders, gently bring your focus back to the breath and back to the counting. Aim to count for at least 10 breaths or for as long as you feel comfortable.

4–7–8 breathing

To do this breathing technique, sit or lie down comfortably and place the tip of your tongue against the roof of your mouth, just behind your front teeth. Close your mouth and inhale quietly through your nose for a count of four. Pause at the top of your inhale and hold your breath for the count of seven. Then, when you are ready, exhale slowly and completely through your mouth for the count of eight, making a whooshing sound as you release. Repeat the cycle a few times to help relax and calm your mind.

Parasympathetic activation breathwork

Parasympathetic breathing involves making your exhale longer than your inhale to activate the body's relaxation response. To practise this, find a quiet and comfortable place. Close your eyes or lower your gaze and begin to breathe. Inhale slowly and deeply through your nose for the count of four. Pause at the top of your in-breath for a moment, then, when you're ready, exhale slowly and completely through your mouth for a count of six to eight seconds. Repeat this breathing pattern for several minutes, focusing on extending and relaxing your exhale. As you continue, try to make your exhales even longer, gradually increasing the exhale-to-inhale ratio.

A regular pranayama practice can stimulate the parasympathetic system, countering the overstimulation that our bodies go through during the fight or flight response. It also acts as the gateway into our soul – our sanctuary for peace.

CHAPTER 8

SOUL EXPANSION AND AWAKENING TO YOUR SOUL'S SCRIPT

Are you living your life in alignment with your soul's script? Is the true essence of you being expressed and shared or repressed and ignored? Are you allowing your soul to light up? Let's explore.

I believe that our soul, the consciousness behind our skin, came here to expand towards its higher seat of self and source. It chose your body as its vessel in which to journey through life on this earth. It came here to live through all it needs to, in order to transcend its human limitations, egoic thoughts and restrictive habits, and grow full in light and love. Your soul will be put through its paces, it will face adversity and challenge, in order for you to dig deep and find your truth. Have you heard the saying 'Pain is inevitable, but suffering is a choice'? When we allow the soul to expand and awaken, we go through a maturation process where we realise that to stay stuck in the pain is ineffectual – it is not what the soul desires. The soul teaches us the importance of transcending this place of pain by shifting focus to a place of power and love. **When your soul is awakened and you are in tune with its calling, you are set free.**

When we shift our perspective to view every interaction in life as an opportunity for growth and expansion, it can be easier to navigate the changes that come our way. I often refer to this as the gift within the struggle. Surrendering to this reality can be difficult at first because when you are in the middle of challenge and struggle it can be hard to comprehend, understand or believe that there is a lesson, gift or silver lining to this situation. Often when in this place, it is raw, it's painful, it can appear like hell. However, if we lean into our hearts and listen to our soul, we'll hear a voice that says *I've got you.* We'll feel a hand that, reaches out to hug and hold us. We'll sense a knowledge that no matter what the outcome, it will be OK. From this place of awareness, we are better equipped to process the experiences that have entangled us. By approaching each moment with openness, we can receive unexpected blessings, and we can trust that behind every struggle lie gifts waiting to be unpacked. Every setback holds lessons that move us towards our soul's freedom and expansion.

As we begin to release from the struggles and strains of life, our soul begins to light up. Then we learn to walk through life with our hearts open to receiving, rather than constricting and closing. **We learn to forgive rather than freeze.** We shed another layer. We no longer stay stuck in the hatred, anger or fear we were once in captivity to. We reconnect with our innermost being and understand the unique script that our soul is meant to follow.

Awakening to your soul's script

The expansion of the soul refers to it growing full in its expression; it involves us going outward shining our light. However, before our soul can be freed to do this, it must first go inward. These two phenomena of the soul expanding and going inward to unite with its inner script and callings are interconnected, but they are distinct when it comes to the journey of the souls awakening. We cannot expand without firstly returning home to our soul. We then take the wisdom from our soul script to guide us on our expansive journey forward.

Soul expansion involves embracing growth, opening up to new perspectives and ideas, stepping outside our comfort zone and seeking evolution. It encourages us to follow our curiosity and cultivate a sense of awe and wonder about the world and ourselves. Awakening to our soul's script, on the other hand, involves going inward. It is about introspection and reflection; it is the art of tuning in to the inner wisdom of our soul's calling. It is where we can uncover our passions and our purpose, and truly listen to the whispers of our soul, to God, the universe or a higher source of power.

The roadmap within

To awaken our soul's script, we must focus on going inward, back home to the source. This requires you to land softly into your heart, to allow it to open and to be graciously guided by your higher self. It is a journey of surrender and trust, of letting go of control and allowing the universe to guide you towards your highest good.

It involves three main steps: *Connecting* to your soul script, *Listening* to your soul's guidance, and *Aligning* with your soul's purpose.

1. Connecting to your soul script

In order to connect with your soul script, you must first silence the mind, reduce the distraction and chaos from the physical world, and create a safe space to go within. This may involve practices such as meditation, journalling or spending time in nature. By quietening the mind and tuning into your soul's voice, you can hear its whispers and discover your path and unique script.

2. Listening to your soul's guidance

Once you have established a connection to your soul, you must then trust the guidance that you receive. Our souls are constantly trying to communicate to us through intuition, signs, nudges, synchronicities and by leading us to experiences that will help us to grow. By allowing this navigational light beam to guide us, we can navigate life's challenges with more grace and wisdom.

3. Aligning with your soul's purpose

I believe each of us is born with a unique purpose. Awakening to this purpose involves uncovering our talents, gifts, passions, values and aligning our actions and behaviours to that which truly fuels our soul. When we live in alignment with this source script, we can experience a life of more joy, fulfilment and inner peace, knowing that we are living authentically.

In a world that often values external success and validation, it is easy to lose sight of our own soul script. I truly believe, however, that if we awaken to our soul script and live in alignment with our purpose, we can transcend much of the struggle and pain in our lives.

Take the example of a lady who attended one of our Soul Space retreats a few years ago. She had been working in the corporate world in a high-stress job for many years and was now feeling burnt out and disconnected. After spending a couple of days immersed in meditation and quiet reflection, which allowed her time to connect with her innermost self and her soul's calling, she realised that her true passion lay in healing practices and yoga, and that she wanted to create a space where others could come to heal and find peace. After the retreat, she decided that she would now align with her soul's script and take action. She began upskilling and retraining in certain areas of health and healing and eventually left her corporate job. She since has gone on to set up her own beautiful studio space and community where she offers classes, workshops and retreats focusing on mindfulness, healing and self-care. Through connection, listening and aligning with her soul's calling, she has found a deep sense of fulfilment and purpose in her life.

Journalling prompts

Prompts to connect to your soul's script

Reflect on a time when you felt a strong sense of intuition. What were the circumstances surrounding this experience and what did it reveal to you about your soul's script?

What brings you joy and fulfilment in life? Reflect on moments when you feel most alive and connected to your true essence.

What values are most important to you?

What practices or rituals help you connect with your higher self and expand your awareness? How can you incorporate more of these practices into your daily life?

Explore your dreams and aspirations. What does your soul yearn for at this moment in your life? How can you align your goals and intentions with your soul's deepest desires?

Pay attention to signs and synchronicities in your life. What messages might the universe be trying to communicate to you about your soul's path and purpose?

Do you practise self-love and self-care to nurture your soul? How can you create a sacred space within yourself to listen to the wisdom of your soul?

Prompts for your soul's expansion

Reflect on past challenges or setbacks. How have these experiences shaped your soul's evolution and growth? What lessons have you learned from these obstacles? What were the gifts that were waiting for you behind the shadows?

Consider the relationships in your life. Are there any that are not serving your soul's growth and expansion? How can you create healthy boundaries and cultivate connections that support your soul's journey?

What fears or doubts are holding you back from expanding your inner essence and your soul? What is stopping you from standing in your light? Who or what is dimming your light right now? How can you work through these fears and blockages to move and expand forward?

Reflect on moments of joy, passion and inspiration in your life. How can you cultivate more of these 'glimmer' moments to foster your soul's expansion?

Visualise the highest, most radiant, purest version of yourself, fully embodying your potential, your purpose and your soul's script. How can you align your thoughts, actions, beliefs and behaviours to support this vision of your soul being free and expanded?

Take a moment to pause and connect with your innermost guidance, wisdom and intuition. What messages or insights are coming to you in this moment? What does your soul need to do in order to expand for your highest evolution and liberation?

What one thing can you do for your soul that will allow you to step bravely into your light and enable you to sing from your soul's script?

By engaging with these journalling prompts, you can deepen your understanding of your soul's script and take meaningful steps towards aligning with your highest purpose and potential. Embrace the journey of self-discovery and transformation and allow your soul to awaken to the beauty and truth of who you are.

The ripple effect

When you throw a pebble into a pond, the ripples fan out over the water. There is peace and stillness in the water until it is disrupted by the pebble. The pebbles in our life are usually all the things that cause us stress and distraction, pulling us away from living from a soul-centred space.

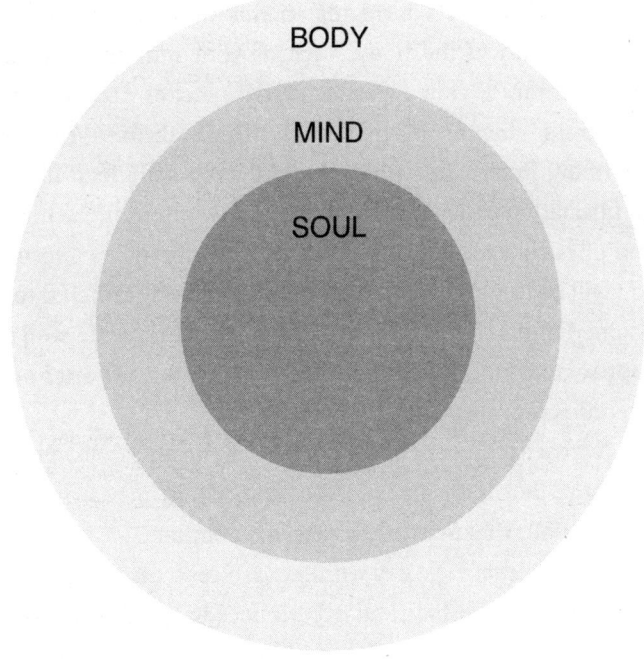

On the flip side, if you can imagine your soul, the essence of who you are is in the centre, and fanning out from this are your mental energies (thoughts, emotions, feelings) and then your physical body (cells, organs, blood, tissue, bones). Your soul is constantly signalling information to your body via the emotional realm. If your soul is vibrant and activated, it will send empowering, uplifting and peaceful ripples outwards to your mental energies and on to your body. You will be in a state of harmony, where everything is in flow.

However, if your soul is squeezed, suppressed and smothered, it cannot send out its ripples of light and love into the mind. Therefore the mind becomes agitated, anxious and clogged and you end up living a path that's not truly connected to your soul. This interference sends distress signals to the body, resulting in dysregulation of the nervous system. When the nervous system is dysregulated, this impacts all the major functionalities of the body, such as your immune system, your hormones, your digestive system, etc. as discussed in the stress chapter of this book. These distress signals, stemming from a squeezed or suppressed soul, lead to the manifestation of negative thoughts and emotions in the mind and physical symptoms or ailments in the body. As a result, you will be out of balance, your mind and body tethered to a strained and squeezed soul. **Ultimately, when your soul is suppressed, your mind becomes depressed, and your body becomes repressed.**

A great example of this is the Russian nesting dolls, where the large doll is on the outside, and within this are many smaller dolls that fit neatly inside one another. This is similar to the layers that we carry within ourselves – all the different emotions and traumas and experiences in our life. It is also symbolic of the soul that lives within the mind, and the mind within the body. If the soul is crying inside, if the soul is unhappy, it feeds energy to the mind and into the body.

Think about two identical twins. Twin A is carefree and joyous, always radiating positivity and happiness. She's in a loving marriage and she approaches life with a sense of fun and ease, allowing herself to fully experience and enjoy each moment. While she may not adhere to the healthiest of life-style habits, she doesn't stress, her soul is at peace and she is content with who she is. In contrast, Twin B is meticulous about her health and her appearance and constantly worrying about her diet, her exercise regime and how she is perceived in the world. She's in an unloving marriage that is quite toxic, and despite her efforts to maintain good physical health, her stress, anxiety and perfectionism weigh heavily on her soul.

Who do you think is the healthiest? Twin A. This high-lights the importance of nurturing a peaceful and happy soul as a vital component of good health. We can only come back into alignment when we allow ourselves time and space for the soul to be heard. **Our soul is an integral part of our inner pharmacy. A happy soul is the foundation of good health.**

Reflection: are you living in alignment with your soul's whispers?

It's important that we learn to pause and reflect so that we can hear the essence of who we are, we can hear the whispers of the soul. It's important that we start to prioritise things in our lives that bring us alive. So pause for a moment and consider the following reflective questions.

* What brings you peace? Do you have enough peace in your life?

* Do you trust in the universe or God? What daily practices can you implement to help bring you closer and deeper into your soul and to a place of inner ease and calm? Write about this and commit to one small practice each day to help you align with this mission.

* What brings your soul alive? Draw a picture or write about a time in your life when you felt fully alive, invigorated, free. Where were you? Who was in your life? What were you doing? Take time to write about this and ask yourself, *What is it in life that truly brings me alive?*

Where science meets spirituality

Believe it or not, some of the main chakra positions bear an extraordinarily close resemblance to the nervous system. Chakras are energy centres in the body that spin like wheels, allowing for the flow of energy or prana. There are seven main chakras all located along the spinal column from the base of the spine to the top of the head, which resembles that of the nervous system (spinal column and the brain). These chakras play a crucial role in maintaining the balance of energy in our physical, mental, emotional and spiritual bodies. Each chakra is connected to specific organs, emotions and attributes, and when these energy centres are balanced and harmonised, we experience optimal health and wellbeing.

The nervous system contains what we call plexuses, while the energetic system contains chakras. Chakras and plexuses are different forms of energy systems. Plexuses are networks of nerves and blood vessels in the physical body, while chakras are part of the subtle body. Interestingly, the locations and connections of these plexuses to vital organs align with the body's chakra system:

* Root chakra (Muladhara): sacral/coccygeal nerve plexus

* Sacral chakra (Svadhisthana): sacral nerve plexus

* Solar plexus chakra (Manipura): celiac (solar) plexus

* Heart chakra (Anahata): cardiac plexus

* Throat chakra (Vishuddha): pharyngeal plexus

* Third Eye chakra (Ajna): carotid plexus, pineal gland, optic nerves

* Crown chakra (Sahasrara): cerebral cortex.

It's fascinating to think how ancient spiritual beliefs about chakras may have unknowingly aligned with the complex network of nerve pathways in the body, shedding light on the interconnectedness of everything – the physical body and the energetic body.

Soul craft

Your soul craft is the unique talent, passion or creative pursuit that brings you joy and fulfilment and that is aligned to your inner soul script. When you craft a life that aligns with your soul, you live authentically and with greater peace. Each person's soul craft is unique, so creating your own personal WHY and PATH is essential in order to live your authentic life.

Understanding your WHY and designing your own PATH

These are powerful written exercises that you might need to do a few times to find your goal, or it might come in a flash of lightning. Please also be aware that your WHY might change depending on which season of life you are in. Dig in and explore

What is your WHY?

∗ What are my dreams, desires and soul whispers?

∗ How do I show up for myself and my beliefs daily? How do I continue to keep people and things in my life that nourish me? How do I come home to my heart's desire every day so that I can stay aligned with my dreams, passions and purpose?

∗ Yielding authenticity; yearning for greatness. By listening to your soul and being truthful to your desires, you begin to live authentically. How can you keep surrendering and letting go of what no longer serves you so that you can liberate your soul and live with more ease, love, joy and grace?

Take some time to contemplate these powerful questions, sitting in silence or with some nice background music, to bring awareness and connection from your soul's self (energetic self) to your human self (physical self).

What is your PATH?

∗ Personal goal and intention. Set a goal or intention that you want to achieve. Be specific. See this vision/picture. Start the journey.

∗   **Aligned focus.** Every day, choose at least one thing that will keep you focused on this goal. Choose people, places and things that will inspire you to stay aligned with the intention.

∗   **Truth and trusted commitment.** Share your vision with trusted colleagues, friends and family who will keep you inspired and aligned to your desire. Be truthful with yourself. Back yourself and keep believing in your capabilities. Trust your heart's desire to achieve this outcome. **I believe God or the universe only places into your heart that which you are destined to fulfil.**

∗   **Honour your journey.** As you make progress, remember to honour each step with an open heart and a humble acknowledgement of your achievements.

Please take as much time as you need to reflect on and contemplate these questions and see what insights and answers surface for you.

CHAPTER 9

HOW TO LIGHT UP YOUR SOUL: THE 11 PILLARS

There are 11 pillars to help illuminate and light up your soul, and we will explore them all below:

1. Overcoming the 'not enough' syndrome

2. Surrendering – the freeing power of letting go and letting flow

3. Coming home – living authentically, owning your truth, honouring your soul

4. The power of pause

5. Self-compassion – embracing yourself with kindness

6. Soulful connections – nurturing connectivity and community

7. Laughter – lighten up

8. Soul recharge – unplug to reconnect

9. Soulful serenity – harnessing the healing power of nature

10. Illuminating the soul – igniting inspiration, passion, purpose and meaning

11. Letting the divine grace flow.

1. 'Not enough' syndrome

This is a journey I have been on and one that I continue to grow through year on year. I've done a lot of work on this area in my life, but I know I am not a masterpiece. I'm still a work in progress, as I believe we all are. **We're all elegantly flawed in this tapestry of life.**

I believe at the very core of the human spirit lies peace, joy and feelings of being enough. Just like the sky, it is infinite and naturally at ease. What disrupts the peace are the things we let enter into this spaciousness, such as thoughts that can become destructive and negative. These unloving thoughts are like clouds that come and crowd out the natural blue sky. They can block the sun, creating a dullness in the sky, or even become aggressive and crash, creating thunder and lightning storms that disrupts the natural peacefulness of the sky. The same can occur within our minds. These 'clouds' breed inferiority, self-doubt and feelings of not being enough. But beneath all of this chaos lies pure poten-tiality and love. We just need to clear away the clouds and dial down the noise in order to let our divine essence, our soul, be heard and felt again.

The 'not enough' syndrome refers to a mindset or a belief that you are not good enough, worthy enough or deserving enough to go after what you want. It can manifest as feelings of insecurity, self-doubt or inadequacy and it might lead to self-sabotaging and self-punishing behaviours. It stems from negative beliefs about our abilities and a lack of confidence. Are you familiar with inner narratives such as:

* 'I'll ask that guy out when I lose five pounds.'

* 'I'll go for that job when I've another course done.'

* 'I'll never be able to reach my goals.'

* 'I don't deserve to be happy.'

* 'I never measure up to others' expectations.'

* 'I'm a constant failure; I'm always messing things up.'

* 'I'm so stupid. Why can't I do anything right?'

* 'Why did you say that? You're such an idiot.'

* 'I'm not talented enough or smart enough to pursue my passions.'

* 'I'm not thin enough, fit enough or attractive enough.'

* 'I don't have enough money, resources or opportunities to achieve my dreams.'

The roots of the 'not enough' syndrome

Who am I not good enough for?

First, who do you feel you're not good enough for? Is there a voice playing in your mind from early childhood? Did a parent, sibling, teacher, caregiver or coach say something to you? Did somebody at some stage of your life say something that just stuck, and so you were led to believe that is just 'the way you are'? This voice or comment took root in your subconscious mind, and when we are young, our logical brain isn't developed enough to decipher whether this voice is real or not, so we believe it to be the truth.

The imprints

Feelings of not being enough can often stem from our past imprints – past experiences, beliefs or messages that have shaped our self-perception and contribute to feelings of inadequacy. For example, comparison to others, such as your siblings or peers, might have led to a sense of inferiority or jealousy. Rejection or abandonment can create a cascade of fear leading to feelings of insecurity, disconnectedness and being unlovable. Similarly, societal or cultural expectations impose certain ideas of beauty, success or even happiness, which can lead you to believe that you fall short of these standards. This then breeds feelings of not being enough, isolation and imposter syndrome. All of these can leave imprints on our heart that can be destructive when it comes to cultivating inner love, harmony and peace.

Deconstructing the 'not enough' syndrome

To let go of the 'not enough' syndrome, we must be willing to transform our feelings of inadequacy. **We need to step out of** the shadows of niceness and into the beauty of realness; saying 'no' is also love.

The six transformational pillars below can help us do that by enabling us to transform our perspective, providing a very practical path to overcoming the 'not enough' syndrome.

1. Comparison → Inspiration

Instead of using comparison as a way of measuring your worth or abilities, which generates emotions of shame, lack and limitation, turn that energy into a source of motivation by focusing on inspiration. 'Inspiration' means to 'breathe in spirit', to breathe in creativity, to breathe in new life-force energy. When we approach comparison with an attitude of inspiration, we can view it as an opportunity for learning and self-improvement. Instead of viewing others as competition, which breeds jealousy, you can see them as a source of guidance. A beautiful phrase that my husband uses is 'If not you, then who?' If they can do it, so can you.

If you find yourself scrolling on social media and falling into comparison mode, press the pause button. Just press pause. Then ask, *What's showing up for me here? Is there jealousy? Is there bitterness? Am I happy for that person? Am I not happy for that person? And why is that?* Cultivating aware-ness is key. Then you can try to figure out what you want to do with it. What is your choice here? Feel inadequate and deterred or see them as a source of inspiration? Know that if that person can do it well, so can you. Maybe that person will be a shining light for you. There are infinite opportunities for us all in this universe.

2. Judgement → Acceptance and acknowledgement

For a long time, I feared leaving pharmacy. I feared going out on my own, I feared self-employment, because I felt I'd be judged. What would my parents think about me leaving a good, steady job after putting me through college for five years? What would my peers think? Feeling judged is a very human experience, and it can be paralysing.

The antidote to this is acceptance and acknowledgement. Can you drop into a space of acceptance and then acknowledge where you are coming from? My parents didn't care about what job I was in; all they cared about was if I was happy. Letting go of the perception of who you think you should be and accepting yourself as you are will lighten your life. The minute you accept and acknowledge yourself, your vibrational frequency changes and you allow yourself to be liberated.

Passing judgement on others is expensive and destructive.
It drains the heart of vital nourishment
and it expends unnecessary mental energy.
Release yourself from the need to judge yourself and others,
and you will set yourself free of jealousy, of fear, of
comparison, of shame and of blame.
Go freely into your life and into your world,
with an open loving heart,
free from the mental, physical and emotional drainage
that judgement can burden us down with.
We are all beautifully broken.
Embrace your flaws,
shine brightly into the world
with all parts of yourself.
Embrace the uniqueness
that makes you come alive and
know that you are enough.

3. Negative self-talk → Compassion

Transforming your negative self-talk into a more compassionate and supportive inner dialogue is possibly one of the greatest things you can do for your health and wellbeing. We discussed this in detail in the Mind section, but dialling down the voice of negativity and dialling up the voice of compassion is key to overcoming 'not enough' syndrome.

4. Integrated wellness → Lifestyle, behavioural changes

If we are not minding ourselves from a physical, psychological and emotional standpoint, it's easy for our nervous system to tip us into a stressed, exhausted and burnt-out state. In that depleted state, we can become enmeshed in lower emotional vibrational frequencies like shame, guilt and despair. This can derail our lifestyle habits, leading us to eat junk foods, not exercise, spend too much time on screens and not get enough fresh air. In this state, the 'not enough' syndrome thrives.

We all have days and weeks where we might steer off course, but in the grand scheme of things, if we look at lifestyle as medicine, as a guide for behavioural change, this can be a magic tool for deconstructing the 'not enough' syndrome, yielding a life where we feel better, and have more confidence and feelings of worthiness and deservability.

5. Imposter syndrome (the shadow self) → Understanding and empathy

Imposter syndrome is a persistent belief that we are a fraud or we do not belong. We feel we'll be exposed for not being enough. This can be devastating for a lot of people: it can stop them pursuing life, relationships, careers and their dreams. The reality of being human is that we will always find a reason that will stop us, so to overcome this we just need to take one step forward at a time and trust ourselves. We must dissolve the need to control and release the expectation of the outcome. That's really what holds us back – the fear of failure. But what if it works out? Release the fear of the outcome, release the fear of failure, and just give it a go. No regrets.

6. Suppression of emotions ⟶ Release of emotions

I saved this pillar to last, because it's one of the most powerful – I've seen the power it has in my own life and in my work with others. It involves feeling, facing and releasing emotions. To do this, you can create 'mindful me' moments where you scan through what's going on in your life, your body and your emotional world, allowing it to surface and then be released in a healthy way. **The emotions of the soul are held in the body, so let the body speak.**

If we suppress a challenging emotion, it generates more power. It's like a parasite that feeds on the suppression. You have two options here: you either deny the emotion and let it get bigger and thicker, or you can say hello to the emotion and let it out.

How do we meet the emotion? How do we bring it out? Through compassion, patience and knowing that it's a process. There is no green juice that will eradicate a toxic self-image. There is no multivitamin that's going to take this away. We can only deconstruct these emotions through daily and lifelong practices like acceptance, acknowledgement, understanding, implementing lifestyle as medicine, 'me time' moments, mirror work, breathwork, meditation, community, connection, knowing that to be human is to be imperfect, and to be imperfect is to embrace all of yourself.

Practical ways to break through the barrier of not feeling enough

* **Daily affirmations and mirror work:** Look in the mirror and say whatever affirmations resonate with you in that

day: *I am enough. I am willing to love myself. I am willing to release the fear. I am willing to care for myself today.*

* **Self-care:** Set aside time each week where you can do things for yourself. For example, *I'm going to have a bath on a Wednesday night. I'm going to go to yoga class on Tuesday. I'm going to meet up with a friend.* It can even be tiny things such as *I'm going to listen to nice music tonight.* Be consistent and don't let yourself off the hook.

* **Love notes to yourself:** If the thought of writing a 'love note' to yourself makes your skin crawl, simply call it a note. It can be transforming to regularly hear that you're doing a good job and that you're a good person. So write a love note (or send a text) to yourself or pick a buddy and agree to send one to each other once a month.

* **Develop the art of not giving a shit (in a loving, compassionate way):** Let's face it, if you're a sensitive soul like me, not giving a shit doesn't come easily. However, life's not all rainbows and roses, and we do need to learn to let certain things wash away. We must learn to let go of unnecessary stress, to not sweat the small stuff, and instead focus on what truly matters in our life. We must tend to the calling of our soul and not get derailed by the voices or opinions of others.

* **Just take a minute:** The power of 60 seconds can be gamechanging. A minute to dial down the stress, the noise, and cultivate more calm. A minute to breathe deeply when you're in the shower, while waiting in a queue, before you open your laptop, before you close the laptop at the end of the day, before you go to sleep.

* **Accomplishment boards:** Create a board with some pictures of you that you're proud of. When I left pharmacy and we moved to Dublin, I went through a really anxious time. Everything was new to me and I felt inadequate. Gerry encouraged me to make a slideshow using images of things I had done recently that I was proud of. I watched this slideshow every morning. It was only two minutes long, but it was powerful. It was like a little pat on the back to help me keep moving forward, to keep the faith.

* **Friday wins:** Every Friday, reflect back on the mini wins of the week. The idea is to celebrate your successes each week to build greater confidence and soul strength.

2. The freeing power of surrendering

I believe surrendering is not a deep collapsing.
It is not a quitting, or an inability to cope.
I believe it to be something quite different.
To surrender is to humbly bow to your vulnerabilities.
It is the softening into your strength.
It is the dissolving away of your anger, judgement,
shame or blame
And the melting away of external barriers, the dissolution
of the walls of protection that we often uphold or
barricade around us to keep our demons locked in and
love shielded out.
I believe surrendering is the letting go of resistance and
the grip of control or the need to own.

It is the delicate landing and arriving into – who you are
and the acceptance of where you are in this moment.

Surrendering is the spaciousness that allows all the home truths to be seen, heard and felt.
To surrender is to wave the white flag to the peace that resides within.
Surrendering is to come home to your authentic self.
To surrender is to come home.

I wrote this piece one day when I was experiencing a great shift in my life, when I felt I was shedding the old Miriam, the version of myself I thought would be seen and appreciated. As I look back on my journey, I realise that surrendering has been a constant companion in my life. It has been the greatest of the lessons that I have learned and relearned in various aspects of my existence: from relationships to career choices, from motherhood to personal growth, surrendering has been both my greatest adversary and my greatest teacher.

There have been many times in my life where I have had to sit deep into my meditation practice to find my life's true path. The most aligned decisions are not necessarily the easy ones. They require you to stretch beyond your comfort zone and break past limiting beliefs. Often these decisions may seem wrong at first, because you think, *Shouldn't it be easy to follow my soul's calling? Shouldn't it bring me into flow state and make me feel happier and content?* The answer is yes and no! It's like the metamorphosis of a caterpillar into a butterfly. The caterpillar feels safe as it is, familiar in its surroundings, knowing no better until its evolution begins. When the caterpillar forms its chrysalis, it is caged within a dark space, the unknown. But out of this dark space of introspection, reflection and fear emerges a magnificent butterfly. Perhaps you're in a relationship or a career and you feel like the caterpillar – your environment is safe, steady, familiar, but deep down you know it's lacking something. Your soul knows there's something deeper within that needs to be expressed and explored, so you leave the relationship or the job, and in those early days it is raw and painful. You are now in the chrysalis of your transformation. And with time, trust and patience, you come out the other side with greater clarity, freedom and a new era for your soul's evolution.

The very act of surrendering allows for a freedom, a dropping into the heart and a trust that everything will turn out as it is meant to. **Surrendering is a powerful strength that comes when we let go of trying to attain the impossible.**

We always mourn losing a past version of ourselves. Transition involves finding a balance between letting go and inviting in.

A rebirthing process

I have gone on this metamorphosis journey many times in my life and I wouldn't change any of it. Most recently, stepping into the role of motherhood has been life-changing. It is beautiful but challenging at the same time. It brought me on a rebirthing process of my innermost self. In my experience, you are forever changed when you become a mother. My priorities changed, my life's direction transformed, my heart opened more than ever before. I initially thought I could 'do it all'! I thought I could be a full-time mom, run my own business, keep all the balls in the air. The overwhelming responsibility and constant demands of caring for two young children while trying to navigate my career forced me to ask deeper questions about myself and the life I wanted to lead. Surrendering made me sit deep in my heart and ask some humbling questions, like:

* What do I need to let go of?

* What do I need to surrender to?

* Who or what type of person do I need to surrender into or let go of?

With the help of Brighid, my psychotherapist, and my own meditation practice, I could hear the whispers, I could sense the nudges. The answer became clear and so simple: I needed to let go of fear and embrace love. I needed to let go of expectations and trust in the wisdom of the soul. I knew I couldn't be 'the dentist with the rotten teeth', telling people to take care of themselves, to follow their heart and live a life that is aligned to their truth if I wasn't doing that myself. So, I let go of a lot of jobs, I said no to a lot of stuff, but I knew deep in my heart where I needed to be and, more importantly, where I desperately *wanted* to be. My kids are my whole world, and I knew that I would never get those early formative years back. I could feel my heart bursting when I thought about being home with them. The tightness and knots in my chest and tummy softened, and relief spread across my shoulders when I thought of stepping back from work and stepping into my role as a stay-at-home mother. I knew I had to surrender to the here and now, and design my life around supporting the needs of myself, my family and my home. I needed to let go of my need to control everything and be perfect. I had to surrender to the vulnerability of not having all the answers and to making mistakes. I had to surrender to the chaotic but beautiful journey of motherhood, the job that has no job description, only to be present as much as you can, show love and keep breathing!

I had to learn how to surrender the 'I can do it all' disease because it comes at a severe cost – this cost often manifesting as a breakdown in something, a severing in your relationship with yourself, your partner or kids, or a breakdown in your health. It has been and continues to be a humbling experience, a recognition that true strength lies in vulnerability, in asking for help, acknowledging my limitations and listening to my heart. It has deepened my faith and encouraged me to trust that we are always being guided and supported, even in our most challenging situations.

It is imperative that we learn how to surrender, that we learn that the act of letting go is for the sake of our evolution and is needed to allow our souls to expand. We must let go time and time again; we must lean into the callings of our soul and into the rawness of how uncomfortable these decisions can make us feel. **But remember, beyond the cocoon phase of metamorphosis lies liberation and freedom, where you fly into a life of new beginnings and new opportunities.**

Surrendering is not the end; it is a new beginning. It is a journey that requires trust, patience and an open heart. It is a gateway to a deeper understanding of ourselves and the world around us. It is a path to freedom and fulfilment.

The challenges of life occur so that we learn to release the need to know or control or even understand.
In the uncertainty of life, we must learn to surrender the ego. To trust in a higher source and to just be.

Learning to surrender

* **Acknowledge your feelings:** Allow yourself to feel and process any emotions that come up when thinking about surrendering or what you need to let go of. It's okay to feel sad, angry or hurt.

* **Practise self-compassion:** Be kind to yourself and recognise that letting go is a process. It's normal to struggle when you are letting go of something that has been part of your life for a long time.

* **Let go of control and have faith:** Surrendering means recognising that we don't always have control over every situation. Allow yourself to let go of trying to control everything and trust in the process – this requires **trusting in a higher power.** If you believe in a higher power (God, the universe, angels, higher source, nature or whatever resonates with you), surrendering to that power can help you feel supported and guided through difficult times.

* **Meditation, breathwork and prayer:** These practices bring you graciously into the present moment and allow for greater acceptance of things as they are, helping to alleviate stress and promote a sense of peace.

* **Release expectations and attachments:** When you let go of expectation, everything changes. The pressure falls away and a sigh of relief floods the body. Who says you're meant to live a certain way with a certain person in a certain place? If you can surrender to not having any expectations and just let life play out as it is meant to, and if you can let go of attachments to outcomes and embrace the idea that everything happens for a reason, the freeing power of this is truly amazing. Surrendering to the flow of life brings a wonderful sense of peace and acceptance.

* **Seek community and support:** If you are struggling to surrender, seek support from friends, family or a therapist who can guide you through the process. Community breeds a sense of a tribe, which generates feelings of

safety. You will only surrender and truly 'drop' when you feel held and safe.

* **Practise gratitude:** Focus on the positive aspects of your life and practise gratitude for the good things. This can help you shift your perception of the process of surrendering as being weak or negative to seeing it as a positive gateway for new beginnings and opportunities.

Reflective questions

Set aside a few minutes and put pen to paper to answer these reflective questions to help you soften into the process of surrendering:

* Who do I need to surrender my expectations of in order to have more authentic and fulfilling connections?

* What limiting beliefs or patterns do I need to let go of in order to embrace the art of surrendering?

* Who do I need to surrender into or what do I need to melt away in order to create a life of more ease and fulfilment?

* What do I need to let go of; what aspects of myself, my mindset, my habits, my behaviours do I need to release with love?

Reflect on past experiences or challenging times when you surrendered, when you got through it and are now more resilient as a result. Use these as reference points to show that you can do challenging things, that you can get through stressful situations, and that you can come out the other end with greater awareness, clarity, confidence and trust.

Breathwork practice: the surrendering sigh

An audio recording in which I guide you through this meditation can be found at www.soulspace.ie/lightup with the password LIGHTUP.

Follow the guide below to do this breathwork exercise while using the mantra *I let go, I surrender.*

Find a quiet and comfortable place to sit or lie down. Take a few long, deep breaths to relax your body and mind. Inhale deeply through your nose, and on your inhale say in your mind *I,* and as you exhale, let out a long, slow sigh and say in your mind *let go.* Feel the tension and stress leaving your body with each sigh. You can alternate this with the mantra *I* on the inhale and *surrender* on the exhale. This helps to keep you focused on the act of letting go and surrendering. Repeat the deep inhale and long-exhale sighs for several more breaths, focusing on releasing any negative energy or emotions that may be weighing you down.

Allow yourself to fully surrender to the breath and the present moment, letting go of any worries or burdens. Allow yourself to feel the connection to love in your heart – your soul's presence. With each exhale let your body sink into the holding hands of divine grace, trusting you are exactly where you are meant to be.

After a few minutes, take a moment to rest and allow yourself to feel the effects of the practice on your body, mind and soul. When you are ready, slowly open your eyes and return to your day, hopefully feeling lighter, freer and more at peace.

Every day is a new day. A day where we get to rise up in our own lives. A time to let the old die and let the new be reborn. It's about shedding the old layers so that we can reveal a whole new life inside. Keep shedding and surrendering.

Keep breaking old habits and breaking new ground. Keep reaching inside and releasing that inner new life and spirit that is waiting to shine and come alive.

3. Coming home: living authentically, owning your truth, honouring your soul

Coming home is more than just returning to a physical place; it's about finding your true self, living authentically and honouring the call of your soul. It involves owning your truth, standing up for what matters and listening to your heart, even when that means making tough decisions. Coming home is an inward journey of self-discovery, inner alignment and spiritual awakening.

How do we come home?

Living authentically and owning your truth

Coming home starts with living authentically, being true to yourself and standing firm in your truths, beliefs and values. It means embracing your uniqueness, owning your story and expressing yourself honestly and openly. When you live authentically, you align with your true essence and create a sense of inner harmony and integrity.

Listening to your heart and honouring your soul's calling

Coming home requires listening to the whispers of your heart and following its guidance by regularly pausing, breathing and listening. We can only hear the callings when we get quiet enough to actually hear them, feel them or sense them. We must regularly detach from distraction so that we can truly tune in to our essence. **Your heart holds the keys to your deepest desires and passions, leading you towards a life that is in alignment with your soul's purpose.** The heart is your altar. Connect to it through the breath and kneel before it through prayer. Anchor into its gentleness, for it knows what you need best. Place your hands over your heart, breathe, let your body soften and ask that whatever it is afraid of to be healed. Ask that whatever is hurting be understood. Ask for the courage to move out of the shadows of fear and into the most empowered state of self, which is one of love, freedom, peace and joy.

Asking 'What would love do?'

Love is the most powerful force in the universe, capable of guiding us towards compassion, connection and unity. When faced with difficult decisions or challenges, asking yourself, 'What would love do?' can help you make choices that are aligned with your good nature and the greater good of all.

Bow your head and forgive yourself

Bow your head towards your heart and forgive yourself for all the times you were not able to honour your heart's callings. For all the times you turned your back on your soul. For all the times you criticised yourself. Bow graciously to this altar within your heart space and say, *I'm sorry. I see you. I'm now ready to listen, to feel and to be guided by your whispers.* Tread softly; for you are easing into a new way of living, a rebirthing. Let your tears fall and land softly on your cheeks. Welcome your true self back home into your heart, your mind, your breath and your body.

Journalling prompts and reflective exercises

* What does the deepest essence of me long for? When I take away all external distractions and societal expectations, when I remove the egoic mind and all of the 'should haves'

and 'could haves', what's left? What is my heart yearning for right now?

∗ Did you ever ignore or dismiss your inner wisdom? Reflect on a time when you didn't listen to your intuition and write about the consequences of that decision.

∗ Imagine your ideal life where you are aligned with your heart's calling and inner wisdom. Describe this vision in detail and consider what steps you can take to move closer to this reality.

∗ What fears or doubts are holding you back from following your heart's calling? Explore these limiting beliefs and challenge yourself to reframe them in a more empowering light.

Breathwork practice

To embark on a breathwork practice for tuning into the wisdom of your heart's longing, begin by finding a quiet and comfortable space to sit or lie down.

Turn your gaze inwards, soften your body and breathe. Bring your awareness to the heart space and imagine it softening, releasing and relaxing. As you continue to breathe, let go of any distractions or worries, focusing solely on the rhythm of your breath and the beating of your heart. Begin to repeat to yourself *Dear [your name], the deepest essence of my being, please guide, advise and show me what the next best steps are towards greater peace, joy and fulfilment in my life. Please give me clarity and hope. Please make clear to me what my deepest desires and needs are.*

Trust that within this space of stillness and quiet, you will begin to hear the gentle whispers of your soul, guiding you towards your true purpose and calling. Stay present with your breath and your heart's guidance, allowing any emotions or insights to surface and be acknowledged.

When you feel ready, gently come back to the awareness of your surroundings, carrying with you the clarity and guidance that your heart and soul have provided.

Trust in the power of your breath to connect you to your innermost being and allow this practice to be a source of strength and inspiration as you journey towards fulfilling your deepest desires and dreams.

4. The power of pause

Did you know that giving yourself the gift of pause and rest can have a positive impact on your soul's glow and your overall health and wellbeing? Research shows that periods of rest and relaxation can greatly help reduce stress, improve immune function, lower blood pressure and enhance cognitive abilities. By regularly pausing and giving yourself permission to rest, you are not only taking care of your physical health, but also nourishing your mental and emotional wellbeing. Pressing pause in life's often chaotic world can be such a gift. It gives yourself permission to recharge your batteries and reconnect with your soul. **Rest isn't laziness; it increases productivity.**

Commit to incorporating moments of pause and rest into your daily routines, whether it's a few minutes of deep breathing, sitting in silence to enjoy a cup of tea, popping on your headphones to do a meditation, taking a short nap or simply stepping outside for a breath of fresh air. These small acts of pausing and self-care can have a huge impact on your health and wellbeing.

The gap: the portal home

There is a powerful space between our inhalation and our exhalation. This is the 'gap' or the place of pause, stillness, spaciousness. I use this practice in all my yoga classes to showcase the power of how we can send our intentions out into the universal field, so that we can raise our vibration and manifest that which we desire within our heart space.

As you inhale, you pause at the top of the in-breath. Into this gap you send your intention, your prayer – whatever you're trying to manifest. I visualise this intention entering my energy field so that it then can attract, 'vibe' or connect with the energy in the universe that I'm trying to draw back in. This for me is the powerful portal to manifestation. After this gap, this pause, I exhale and release through a 'surrendering sigh'. At the end of this exhale, again there is a pause, and again into this gap I send my intention.

Sometimes I send what I want to manifest into the gap at the top of my inhale, and send that which I'm trying to let go of, or surrender, into the gap at the end of the exhalation. This is because I believe we can only attract what we want once we have cleared the debris to create space for it. This gap is really where our point of power for manifestation occurs. Through this gap, through this energy, through the spaciousness we expand.

Press pause journalling prompts

* What does 'the power of pause' mean to you? How do you typically react in moments of stress or uncertainty? Do you go into a fight, flight, freeze, fawn, flop or flow state? Consider how pausing could help you to respond instead of react, and how this could more mindfully help you in these situations.

* Identify areas of your life where you could benefit from incorporating more moments of pause. How might taking

intentional breaks throughout your day improve your wellbeing and productivity?

* Imagine a scenario where you are faced with a challenging decision. How could pausing to tune into your intuition and inner wisdom influence the outcome? Can you imagine how the pause can more deeply connect you with your soul's callings and how this can allow you to make decisions that are aligned to your authentic self? Explore the potential benefits of making space for reflection before taking action.

* Experiment with different ways to incorporate pauses into your daily routine, perhaps taking a few deep breaths, practising mindfulness, or simply stepping away from a stressful situation. Reflect on how these pauses affect your mindset and emotional state.

5. Self-compassion as the gateway to inner peace and harmony

You might never know the importance of a kind word, a gentle smile or a random hello ... Don't look for affirmation or approval for your kind acts. Just do them anyway. Why? Because by doing so you are making our world a better place, one interaction at a time.

Embracing self-compassion is a powerful act of kindness towards ourselves. It allows us to acknowledge our own humanity, our truth and even our perceived weaknesses or mistakes. The key, however, is to acknowledge these things without judgement, shame or self-sabotage, and instead explore them with kindness and love, reverence and respect, and a deep understanding of our soul's journey.

When we practise the act of self-compassion, we treat ourselves with the same warmth and care that we would offer to a dear friend in need. Remember, you are worthy of your own love and forgiveness.

A truly transformative time in my life was when I embraced the practice of self-compassion through the process of inner child work. For years I had been very hard on myself, but the moment I started to embrace inner child work, everything changed. This process involved speaking to my inner child as if she was still alive within me. I had to bring her everywhere with me, speak with her, ask her what she needed or wanted. I imagined her as a younger version of myself who needed love, care and understanding. I offered her words of comfort and reassurance whenever I felt overwhelmed or anxious; I would tell her that she was loved, valued and worthy, just as she was. I began to embrace my inner child with compassion and kindness, acknowledging her fears and offering comfort and support. I found that by connecting with my inner child, I was able to tap into a wellspring of self-compassion and self-love that I hadn't realised was within me. This stopped me self-sabotaging or punishing myself, as I didn't want to hurt this beautiful little girl. I wanted to be kind to her, to love her, respect her and make her happy.

Fast forward a few years. When I look at my own daughter, the love and adoration I have is indescribable. I now see my inner child in my daughter. Self-compassion changes everything. It brings home a sense of love and wonderment and awe. Instead of hating yourself, you can begin to love yourself. When you create a more loving, harmonious relationship with yourself, your whole life changes. You start saying yes to yourself more, you start honouring your needs, but, more important, you begin to regulate your nervous system and come back into coherence. When the loving and healing emotions of the heart are allowed to flow again, you take yourself out of stress mode and into relaxation and ease mode. This not only makes you feel better, but dramatically uplifts and upregulates your immune system and health. Therefore, compassion = greater health.

Self-compassion, I believe, is one of the most powerful tools to greater health, wellbeing and performance. Self-compassion is not a frailty – it's not a stepping away from or distraction from the truth; in fact, I believe it's the opposite. It's owning up to our vulnerabilities and our mistakes and flaws. It's looking at ourselves in the mirror and straight into our eyes with love and compassion, even when we feel we have done wrong or done something that has not been our best. The moment we see this and offer love and compassion, we develop greater confidence to go forth into the world with honesty, authenticity and benevolence.

How to develop greater self-compassion

Reflective exercises

* Practise writing a self-compassion letter to yourself, acknowledging your struggles, validating your feelings, and offering words of kindness and support. Read this letter whenever self-doubt or self-criticism arises.

* Engage in a loving-kindness/self-love meditation (page 210). Practise this meditation every day for at least a month. By focusing on phrases of compassion and kindness towards yourself, you cultivate feelings of warmth and acceptance

and begin to strengthen your relationship with yourself. This is the precursor to greater inner peace, ease, love and harmony.

* Create a self-compassion ritual or routine that involves self-care activities, such as mirror work, reading, journalling, taking a bath or spending time in nature. Prioritise moments of tenderness and self-nurturing in your daily schedule. By doing this you are signalling to your body, mind and soul that *you matter*, and this compassionate time for self is where all the great healing can occur.

Journalling prompts

* If you were to allow your inner voice to be more compassionate and kind, how do you think this would impact your life? How might you look, feel or behave if your inner thoughts, stories and narratives were supportive, encouraging and uplifting?

* Reflect on a time when you were kind and compassionate towards yourself. What did that experience feel like? How did it impact your wellbeing?

* In what ways do you show compassion towards others? How can you extend the same level of compassion to yourself?

* Are there any beliefs or self-imposed expectations that prevent you being kind and compassionate towards yourself? Reflect on these limiting beliefs and explore healthier alternatives.

Breathwork: cultivating kindness within

An audio recording in which I guide you through this meditation can be found at www.soulspace.ie/lightup with the password LIGHTUP.

To begin, find a comfortable seated or lying position where you can relax. Close your eyes or lower your gaze and take a few deep breaths to settle into the practice. With each inhale, imagine breathing in love, compassion and kindness towards yourself. As you exhale, release any negative thoughts or self-criticism.

As you continue this pattern of breathing, allow yourself to fully embrace your emotions and experiences without judgement. Offer yourself the same level of understanding and empathy that you would give to a loved one in need.

With each breath in, envision filling yourself with warmth, comfort and self-compassion. As you breath in, say *I see you, I feel you, I hear you, I forgive you, I love you.* Feel the love and acceptance coursing through your body, soothing any areas of emotional pain or discomfort.

As you breathe out, say *I let go any shame, blame or hurt, I no longer need to hold you in my body. I release you and let you go with love.*

Continue this practice for as long as you feel necessary, allowing yourself to fully surrender to the healing power of self-compassion breathwork. When you are ready, slowly bring your awareness back to the present moment. Go easy and gently.

6. Soulful connections: nurturing connectivity and community

> *A heart that is open and receptive to love is much more likely to yield a body that is more content and a mind that is more at ease.*

When we feel connected, we feel we belong to a tribe. One of the key benefits of being part of a community is that we feel supported by like-minded individuals, which nurtures our spiritual wellbeing. It creates a sense of solidarity that can be a source of comfort and strength during challenging times, and a source of motivation and inspiration during good times. Community and connectivity offer guidance, empathy, encouragement and hope, which allows you to gain more harmony in your soul.

When you are connected to someone, it deepens your understanding of yourself. Through meaningful conversations, mutual exploration and shared experiences you can gain new perspectives that can help you grow. Being part of a community means you can be heard, seen and feel valued.

In the book *The Hidden Life of Trees: What They Feel, How They Communicate*, Peter Wohlleben explores how trees communicate with each other via their own type of nervous system. Trees in every forest are connected to each other through underground fungal networks. They share nutrients and water through these networks, and also use them as a means to communicate to each other. If a tree is in distress (from drought or disease or an insect attack), it will send out a signal that it is in distress and all the other trees nearby will pick up on this signal and alter their behaviour. They then begin to work together in harmony to send help and support to the distressed tree. For example, when young saplings are in a deeply shaded part of the forest, this network is literally a lifeline for them. If they lack the sunlight to photosynthesise they won't survive; however, big trees, including their parents, pump sugar into their roots through this network, enabling them to survive. Wohlleben likes to say that the mother trees 'suckle their young'. This not only highlights the power of connection and community, but it also shows that when we are distressed our distress signals are sent out to those around us and to the very essence of the vessel within which the soul is living.

True heart connection

True heart or soul connection with another person is one of life's greatest gifts. It is what makes relationships, whether friendship, romance or family, thrive and flourish. Being intimately connected doesn't just mean on a physical level: it involves a bonding of our minds and souls. Seeking out moments of true intimacy can be done by simply looking into one another's eyes, speaking from your heart, sharing your truth and opening yourself up to hearing and feeling the other person's truth, allowing you to experience a deep connection with yourself and with others.

When we are part of a community, our body is flooded with powerful neurotransmitters, predominately oxytocin (our love and connection hormone) and serotonin (our happy hormone), which we mentioned in the Body section.

Last year my father faced a very serious illness, which left him hospital-bound for months. He has since, thankfully and miraculously, recovered, but I really believe one of the key foundations that enabled him to recover was the outpouring of love and support he graciously received from his family, friends and community. It was nothing short of amazing. I believe that the power of the kindness and generosity he received gave him hope and strength to keep fighting, aiding his recovery and supporting his healing.

Journalling prompts

* Reflect on a time when you felt truly supported by your friends and family. How did their presence and actions make you feel connected and valued?

* Consider the people in your life who lift and light you up and bring positivity into your world. How do you reciprocate their support and show appreciation for their presence in your life?

* Write about a community or a group that you feel deeply connected to. What values and experiences do you share with this community and how does being a part of it light you up?

Practical ways to increase oxytocin and build community

Human connection and contact is so important. Touch, hugs, eye contact and intimacy all raise oxytocin levels. People often say to me, 'I'm not in a relationship' or 'I'm living away from home/away from my family, so I don't get hugs every day. What can I do?' Believe it or not, a really simple way to do this, even though it might sound silly, is to invest in a teddy bear. Get a teddy bear or a hot water bottle or a pet – something that you can literally hold and snuggle. After all, oxytocin is referred to as the 'snuggle hormone'. Get a massage, some reflexology, anything where the body feels touched, held and safe.

As well as physical contact, the following are great ways to increase oxytocin:

* Do random acts of kindness.

* Join a gym or a class, volunteer or join a charity.

* Spend time with loved ones, family and friends.

* Get involved in community events, local fairs, festivals, fundraisers.

* Support local communities – shop and dine locally to get to know the locals.

* Host and attend local gatherings – book clubs, coffee mornings, street parties, movie nights, etc.

7. Lighten up: the importance of fun and laughter for our soul's health

Laughter is often said to be the best medicine, and for good reason. It has the power to uplift our spirits, improve our mood, reduce stress and anxiety, and enhance our sense of wellbeing. When we allow ourselves time to play, laugh and feel that sense of freedom and youthfulness, our soul comes alive.

Laughter has a huge impact on emotional healing and soulful living because it has the power to heal emotional wounds and provide comfort during challenging times. Laughter allows us to enter into the heart space and release pent-up emotions, let go of stagnation and negativity, and cultivate fluidity and flow, allowing joy, compassion, kindness and gratitude to resurface. By embracing laughter as a tool for emotional healing, we can promote a greater sense of optimism, resilience and soul health.

All worries and stresses seem to melt away when we are fully immersed in the pure magic of laughter. That belly laugh not only transforms mood but also connects you to those around you. Sometimes all you need is a good belly laugh to transform your perspective, brighten your day and nurture your soul.

I believe your beauty, your light, your power, your brilliance are strongest when you're filled with laughter and joy. I believe joy comes to us through the divinity of laughter.

Physically, laughter can reduce stress hormones, increase immunity, increase the release of endorphins and increase blood flow, all resulting in a greater state of relaxation in the body. There is no doubt that laughter leads to greater physical and mental health and wellbeing. Watch a funny movie, read a funny book, meet up with friends, go on a date night ... do things that make you smile.

8. Soul recharge: unplug to reconnect

Take time regularly throughout the day to detach from busyness and business and just be.

We must unplug from the external world to truly plug in to our internal world and to truly 'come home' to ourselves. Learning to have healthier relationships with our screens is so important for mental, emotional and physical wellbeing.

There are numerous benefits to technology; it has changed our lives in so many positive ways. However, without balance, overuse or addiction to our screens can become destructive to our wellbeing, leading to excess stress, strain and the pressures of urgency.

Self-enquiry check-in

∗ How many times a day do you pick up your phone, do you think?

∗ Do you bring your phone to the bathroom with you?

∗ Do you read emails/scroll social media while watching TV?

∗ When you're walking down the street or in a queue, are you reading text messages, catching up on emails or sending voice notes?

* When you're eating your dinner, are you on your phone?

The health benefits of unplugging

Improved quality of life
In a study from the University of Maryland, researchers discovered that when students unplugged from technology, they reported an improved quality of life. In the context of this study, an 'improved quality of life' meant that participants spent more time with friends and family, got more frequent exercise and even cooked more often and ate healthier foods. How did all of these lovely changes occur? Less time spent on their phones gave them the 'free' time to spend doing something else.

Improved performance and productivity
A research study from the university of Bergen in Norway found that employees who were able to mentally detach from work during off hours reported higher levels of wellbeing and overall job satisfaction. When people unplug from work-related tasks, such as checking their work email after hours, they feel fresher and more recharged when beginning work the following day. For anyone who has ever experienced burnout at work, this isn't too surprising. We can only do so much for so long before feeling exhausted, and constantly plugging into our screens doesn't help matters.

Improved sleep
Unplugging results in reduced exposure to blue light, which affects our sleep hormone melatonin, therefore increasing sleep quality and quantity.

Enhanced relationships

More time spent having face-to-face contact increases connection, oxytocin and feelings of security and stability.

Reduced stress, anxiety and mental health issues

Less screen time means less time spent comparing yourself to others.

How to unplug

* Schedule some downtime each day to unplug. For example, the first hour of your day, 15 to 30 minutes during your lunch break or after eight o'clock every evening could be tech-free time.

* Switch off notifications to reduce time spent checking your phone.

* Leave work at work: no emails or phone calls outside work hours.

* Create a tech-free zone at the dinner table and in the bedroom.

* Use detach apps such as ClearLock, Quality Time or Moment to monitor time spent online.

* Read offline.

* Involve friends, family and colleagues to encourage and motivate one other. For example, when you meet for dinner or coffee, agree to leave your phones in your bags.

Reflective exercises

* Try a phone-free day. Observe how this impacts your mental and emotional health. Notice what you can achieve without the distraction.

* Start your day by connecting to yourself through meditation, breathing, writing or movement, rather than checking emails or social media. Try this for 30 minutes each morning and notice how it impacts your mental and emotional health.

* Challenge yourself to go for a run or walk without your phone or any music. Just tune into your own breath and let your inner voice of wisdom be heard.

* Challenge yourself to have tech-free zones in the house or office. Notice how this helps to create enhanced communication and connection between you and your loved ones. Write about your experience.

9. Soulful serenity: harnessing the healing power of nature

We often deny ourselves the ability to see the beauty that is all around us. It's in every child, every tree, every star, every sunset, every bird and every smile. We live in a world filled with infinite miracles and magic.

When we immerse ourselves in nature, in the peaceful stillness of a forest or the vast expanse of a mountain range, we come to realise that we are not separate from the world around us but an integral part of a greater whole, united web of existence that stretches far beyond our individual selves.

Through this interconnectedness, we find a sense of love and security that soothes our souls and fills us with a sense of peace. Nature itself becomes a source of comfort and solace, offering us a sanctuary in which to rest and rejuvenate our spirits. How many of us have taken a walk up a mountain or by the sea in times of distress or grief? There is something healing in the sounds of the ocean and the stillness of the forest. We don't even need to know exactly why we gravitate towards places of nature and beauty during these times, all we need to know is that it helps heal a wounded soul.

As we allow ourselves to surrender to the majesty of nature, we feel our souls begin to shine with a light that is radiant and pure. The barriers we have built around our hearts begin to crumble, and we are able to open ourselves up to the abundance that surrounds us. Nature has a way of grounding us and anchoring us back home to our hearts. Nature's beauty is infectious.

When I dive into the icy waters of the sea, I feel a sense of exhilaration and freedom. I instantly feel alive. The salty ocean water washes away any lingering stress or negativity and my soul lights up.

When I doubt myself, when fear kicks in, I take myself to Mother Nature and hope is always restored. She instils me with a quiet confidence. My anxiety is lowered, my worries dissipate, and I am reminded once again that I am connected to something infinite. It allows me to return home to my soul and the feeling of love that resides within.

The ever-changing cycle of growth and decay

The natural dance and rhythm of nature also reminds us that human life is filled with struggle, change and strain, but when we are attuned to the subtle shifts in our environment, we can learn to surrender to the ever-changing cycle of growth and decay. Nothing in nature blooms all year: each flower has a season, a time to go inwards and contract, and a time to blossom and shine. Animals hibernate, birds migrate, leaves fall. We, of course, are similar, even though we often forget it. We feel that we need to be strong all year round, that we should always be on the go. We must realise that we too have seasons in our lives. There are phases when we will need to go inwards, to rest, to be still, to let go. We are called to die several times in our lives – not a physical death, but a spiritual and emotional shedding, a letting go of all the things that no longer serve us. We can then be reborn into a version of ourselves that is more aligned to our soul's calling for this next stage of our life. Some people call this a 'mid-life crisis'; I call it an awakening.

Just like nature, we must embrace these life cycles with grace and trust the process. If we don't surrender to these letting-go seasons, we end up resisting, fighting, struggling and suffering. There is no ease, grace, joy or flow when we are always in battle mode. If we observe the flow of nature we can open up to a greater flow within us. Being in nature brings a sense of calm and clarity that transcends the chaos of everyday life.

So let us immerse ourselves in the soulfulness and divine grace of nature. In doing so, we allow our souls to shine brightly.

10. Soulful living: inspiration, purpose, passion, meaning

In order to live a truly fulfilled and soulful life, I believe our soul needs to be excited, committed, passionate and inspired.

Inspiration is like a spark that lights a fire within us. It is a gift that lifts us up and propels us in the direction of our deepest dreams. It gives us confidence to pursue our passions, to maximise our full potential. Inspiration pokes us from the inside; it emerges from the depths of our soul and lights a light within. **When we are aligned to our true selves and our soul's core values and script, I believe we naturally glow. We naturally 'light up'.**

When was the last time you felt goosebumps rise like exclamation points along your skin, like something inside you was bursting to get out, like your soul was longing to sing? This is inspiration. This is passion. This is purpose. This is soulful living. This is living **in-spirit**, in rhythm with your spirit.

Wear the orange dress

Life can be short and unpredictable, and we only get one shot at it (in this lifetime!). Embracing the full spectrum of life is not a bonus, it is a necessity. If we want to feel fulfilled, we must be willing to show up for ourselves, forgive our past, develop a harmonious relationship with our deepest selves and follow the compass of our soul.

My husband and I have hosted our annual Soul Space flagship event in the National Concert Hall in Dublin, Ireland, over the last number of years. These events have been incredibly uplifting and transformative days where many of the participants' hearts were opened and their souls liberated.

In the lead-up to our last event, I went shopping to find something to wear. There was one dress (an orange dress) that I instantly loved. The minute I put it on, my soul sang. When I looked in the mirror, I felt excited, proud, strong and beautiful. This dress was loud, it was powerful, it was striking.

But as I looked in the mirror, I heard a voice in my head, like a thunderbolt: *That's a bit much, Miriam! It's too bright and too out there. Maybe you're showing a little too much leg, maybe it's not conservative enough.* The ego's critical voice continued to say things like: *How dare you wear something like that? Who do you think you are? You'd be better off going for the more understated navy or black outfits. You don't want to draw too much attention to yourself. You don't want everyone to think that you love yourself.*

I was amazed by the stories that jolted into my mind at that moment. Even though the fabulous shop assistant shared how stunning she thought the orange dress was, I got shy and said, 'I'm not sure. I'll take it along with the navy and the black dresses and I'll try all three of them on at home.'

When I had finished in the shop, I paused and reflected on the experience I had just had. Even though I had done so much work on harmonising my inner voice, it still bounced up to test me. I was, however, very proud that I was able to catch myself and honour this internal tug of war. My heart and soul were telling me one thing – wear the orange dress – and my head was telling me another – stay small, dim your light and hide your beauty from the world.

The night before the event, I had decided on the navy outfit – I wanted to play it safe. However, the next morning, when I was getting ready, something from deep within said, *NO! Don't wear the navy outfit, wear the orange dress!* My husband came into the room as I was scavenging through my shoes to find a pair that would match this orange dress. He asked in a loving but curious voice, 'What are you doing, Miriam?' I said, 'Change of plan, Gerry. I'm listening to my soul. I'm wearing the orange dress!' I knew that the event wasn't about what I wore, it was about what I would say and the energy we would create for everyone, but I had a feeling that my outfit would have an impact on the show.

A couple of hours later, I was standing on the main stage in front of a thousand people in my orange dress and, thankfully, a pair of shoes that matched perfectly, delivering a talk on the topic of listening to your heart, living authentically and coming home to your soul. A choir had just sung 'True Colours', and I was sharing a beautiful piece on embracing all the colours in our life, when words I had not planned to say flew directly from my soul and out of my mouth. I said that life is not a dress rehearsal, so stop playing small, stop hiding in the shadows, stop hiding your dreams, limiting your power or dimming your light. We need to supercharge our soul by listening to its callings, honouring its whispers and then taking action to live our dreams. I stamped my feet on the ground, stretched my arms in the air and said, **'We need to wear the goddamn orange dress.'**

This line stuck a chord with so many people in the audience that I got hundreds of messages afterwards from women saying, 'Thank you for sharing the story about wearing the orange dress. I will no longer live in the shadows and the darkness of my light. I will wear the orange dress!'

The orange dress is a symbol of being willing to stand up and stand out. Orange is a colour that exudes energy, vitality and creativity. It says, *I am here, I am ready*. By 'wearing the orange dress', we are making a statement that we are not afraid to be seen, to be heard and to be fully present in our lives.

Too often, we save our best clothes for special occasions, waiting for the perfect moment to break them out. But the truth is, every moment we are alive is a special occasion. Each breath, each heartbeat, each step on this earth is a gift that should not be taken for granted.

We must not hide our true selves away, waiting for the perfect opportunity to shine. We must embrace our power right now. We must stand tall, stand out and be unapologetically ourselves.

So let us wear the orange dress of life with pride and confidence. Let us embrace every moment, every opportunity and every challenge with courage and determination. Let us show up, stand out and live life to the fullest, in all its vibrant and colourful glory.

Reflective exercises and journalling prompts

Standing out from the crowd and shining your light is not about seeking validation or approval from others. It is about honouring your inner light and allowing it to illuminate the world around you. It's about embracing your uniqueness and letting youself shine brightly for all to see. So wear the symbolic orange dress and watch your courage and confidence grow.

* **Write a letter** to yourself, expressing your fears and doubts about standing out from the crowd and shining your light. Then write a response to yourself, detailing all the reasons why you are unique, special and deserving of love and recognition.

* **Create a vision board** or collage that represents your true self and the qualities you want to showcase to the world. Include images, quotes and words that inspire you to be bold, confident and authentic.

* **Practise positive affirmations** daily to boost your self-confidence and courage. Repeat phrases such as *I am worthy of success and recognition, I shine my light brightly for all to see* and *I am confident in my abilities and strengths.*

* **Take a step outside your comfort zone** by wearing something that makes you feel confident and empowered – like an orange dress! Notice how your posture, attitude and

energy change when you embody that sense of empowerment and self-assurance.

* **Engage in activities** that showcase your talents and
   passions, whether it's performing on stage, speaking in
   public or sharing your creative work with others. Allow
   yourself to be seen, heard and appreciated for the unique
   gifts and qualities you bring to the world.

* **Reflect and/or journal** on past experiences when you
   have stood out from the crowd and shone your light
   brightly. What lessons can you take from those moments
   to inspire and motivate you to continue stepping into
   your power and embracing your true self?

11. Letting the divine grace flow

*Dear God, let there be peace in my heart, hope in my
soul and faith in my journey. Let the darkness reveal
the light and the light reveal the truth. Dear God,
illuminate my life with joy and peace and ignite my
world with grace and ease.*

When I think about letting the divine grace flow, I am always
called back to the energy of Mother Mary. I have always had
a deep connection to her, and her grace is something I
greatly admire.

Her divine grace energy symbolises unconditional love,
compassion, integrity, humility, forgiveness, healing and
compassion. She's often portrayed as symbol of grace and
strength in times of hardship. Her courage and bravery in
the face of adversity serve as an inspiration to us all. Despite

facing numerous challenges and struggles throughout her life she remained calm, steadfast and unwavering in her faith and integrity. During difficult times, her courage and bravery inspire us to persevere through our struggles, trusting that there is always a higher purpose guiding us.

I believe we can all tap into this divine grace energy by opening the heart and connecting to a higher power through practices like prayer, meditation and spending time in nature. I believe that love is the universal energy of grace, and it doesn't just flow through things outside us – it flows through us all. We just have to cleanse the debris that clogs our heart so we can connect to this divinity, let it flow through us and let us live it, breathe it and be it.

Just as Mother Mary was a vessel for the light of God, we too can cultivate a similar openness and receptivity to divine energy. By embodying qualities such as kindness, compassion and selflessness, we create a space within ourselves for the divine light to enter and illuminate our hearts and minds. Mother Mary's unwavering faith and trust in God serve as a reminder that we too can strengthen our connection to the divine by surrendering our ego and allowing ourselves to be guided by higher spiritual truths. By practising humility and openness, we can align ourselves with the flow of divine energy and allow it to work through us for the highest good of all.

In times of darkness or difficulty, I turn to Mother Mary as a source of inspiration and guidance. Her presence reminds me that even in the face of adversity, we can find strength and solace in our faith and connection to the divine.

In times of gratitude, I thank the Lord. In times of despair, faith is my best friend. When I'm scared, I turn to prayer, I surrender to a higher power. The divine grace meditation below can help you with this.

Clean the heart

Cleaning the heart is imperative to connecting with your soul. Imagine your heart as a mirror. If the mirror is dirty, covered in dust and cobwebs, visibility is impaired – you can't see your own reflection. Just as a dirty mirror can obstruct our ability to see ourselves clearly, a heart filled with negative emotions, attachments and external influences can block our connection to our inner self and to the divine.

If you fill your heart with materialistic things you will block yourself from connecting to your soul. Your heart ought to be a place that harbours your core values and your deepest truths.

Whatever your core value is, be it peace, love, truth or graciousness, your heart should be filled with this value, not with things. These external 'things' are extensions of your energetic entanglements with the world – however it is not *you*, it is not your true source, and it surely is not your divine essence.

It is my belief that the soul speaks to us through the emotions of the heart. If the heart is clogged with negativity, it becomes difficult to listen to the guidance of our soul. By clearing our hearts of negative and external influences, we create space for our divine energy to flow freely. Each of us can open up to being a channel for the divine light. It is our birthright to live in this light and shine it brightly.

Unfortunately, the earthly ego often infects us with emotions like jealousy, anger, hatred and shame. By cultivating virtues such as love, compassion and humility, we create a space within ourselves for the light of God or the universe to flow through us. May we seek to be vessels of grace and love, allowing the divine light to guide us on our spiritual journey home.

Divine grace meditation

An audio recording in which I guide you through this meditation can be found at www.soulspace.ie/lightup with the password LIGHTUP.

Begin by finding a quiet and comfortable place to sit or lie down. Close your eyes or lower your gaze and begin to breathe slowly and deeply. Imagine a radiant, bright golden light or energy above you, shining down on you with love and abundance. Feel the warm glow and the peace of this divine grace surrounding you.

As you continue to breathe, bring your awareness into your heart centre. Place your hands upon your heart and feel the warmth and energy that emanates from this space. Visualise the glowing lights now entering into your heart space, connecting you to the divine source of love and grace. Allow this light to fill your entire being, surrounding you with a sense of peace and harmony.

As you breathe in and out, imagine the light expanding and flowing through your body, mind and soul. Feel yourself opening up to receive the blessings and guidance of the divine.

Stay in this state of connection for as long as you need, allowing yourself to be receptive to the grace and love that is always available to you.

When you are ready, slowly open your eyes and carry this sense of connection with you throughout your day. You can return to this meditation whenever you need to reconnect with your heart and the divine grace that it brings. Remember to use this meditation any time you want to supercharge your soul and light yourself up.

Light-up moments for the soul

◊ Engaging in acts of kindness that fill your soul with warmth and love

◊ Watching a beautiful sunrise or sunset

◊ Feeling the warm glow of the sun on your body, hearing the morning sounds of birds chirping, or listening to the sound of waves crashing

◊ Your favourite fresh flowers on your windowsill

◊ Laughing until you cry

◊ Being surrounded by loved ones on a special occasion

◊ A good night out (or in) with loved ones

◊ Fluffy socks, a cosy blanket, a warm fire and your favourite movie

◊ Attending a spiritual retreat or taking part in a meaningful ritual or ceremony that nourishes your soul

◊ Spending time in quiet reflection or meditating to connect to your inner self

◊ Turning your phone off, unplugging from the world and allowing yourself to be off the hook, if only for an hour!

◊ Self-care practices – that hour of yoga, that walk in nature, that swim in the sea

◊ Hugs, cuddles and kisses with loved ones, with pets, with your favourite teddy!

◊ Bedtime stories, hot cocoa, warm milk, snuggles

◊ The freeing power of surrendering and letting go of something that no longer serves you

◊ Sitting in the silence of a church, lighting a candle, saying a prayer, receiving the divine grace of light, love and hope to settle, soothe and connect you to your higher self and source.

YOUR TOOLKIT FOR HARMONISING THE BODY, MIND AND SOUL

Balancing the body, mind and soul is not a one-size-fits-all solution or a quick fix, but rather a holistic approach to jumpstart your system. By incorporating some of the suggestions below, you can help your body, mind and soul return to balance, harmony and cohesion. I hope you will use the weekly schedules below as guiding maps and LIGHT UP protocols to help energise your body, awaken your mind and supercharge your soul.

The body balance

Balancing the body aims to brings harmony within by improving nutrition, reducing stress, supporting the lymphatic system, boosting circulation and enhancing sleep quality. To do this we will engage in four main pillars:

1. Mindful movement to stimulate lymphatic drainage

2. Adopting a nutrient-rich diet to nourish our bodies

3. Implementing stress-reducing practices

4. Prioritising restful sleep for optimal health and performance benefits.

Weekly body balance programme

Here is a sample weekly schedule focusing on movement of the lymphatic system, good nutrition, reducing stress and aiding sleep.

Nutrition:

* Remove alcohol, reduce sugars and processed food.

* Cook at home if and when possible. Remember 'Vitamin H': bring your own lunch, batch cook (cook once, eat twice).

* Eat the rainbow, and eat your greens.

* Eat more plants (fruits, veggies, herbs, nuts, wholegrains, seeds, spices, lentils, beans).

* Stay hydrated.

Physical:

* Engage in some form of movement each day to stimulate the lymphatic system, reduce stress and cultivate greater wellbeing.

Reduce stress:

* This week, prioritise your own needs and self-care.

* Say no if and when you need to.

* Listen to your heart more and make choices that will bring you more peace and ease.

Better sleep:

* Prioritise better-quality and -quantity sleep by being more mindful of the choices you make that are impacting it.

* Reduce stress, caffeine, stimulants.

* Create a better bedroom environment.

* Go to bed at the same time each night.

* Create a simple night-time routine.

* Change your sheets.

Day 1

* Morning: Start the day with a brisk walk or gentle yoga session to stimulate the lymphatic system.

* Nutrition: Focus on hydrating foods like cucumber, watermelon and leafy greens. Drink plenty of water throughout the day.

* Stress reduction: Practise deep-breathing exercises or meditation for at least 10 minutes.

* Sleep aid: Establish a bedtime routine with calming activities like reading or listening to music before bed. Remove TV or screens for at least one hour before bed.

Day 2

* Movement: Practise heel drops (see page 88) to further stimulate lymphatic flow (this can be done sitting down or standing up).

* Nutrition: Include foods rich in antioxidants like berries, leafy greens and nuts. Make every meal you eat today colourful, with wholesome and nutrient-dense foods. *Cut out all processed foods today.*

* Stress reduction: Do 5–10 minutes of mindfulness – slow everything down today. Slow down how you eat, how you walk, how you talk.

* Sleep aid: Go to bed 15 minutes earlier than usual.

Day 3

* Movement: Practise bouncing up and down on your toes for five minutes or rebounding on a mini trampoline. Shake the body out, shake your arms, your legs. Put on some nice uplifting music and shake, dance and bounce. This will specifically target the lymphatic system.

* Nutrition: Focus on nourishing foods, herbs and spices like cruciferous vegetables, garlic, ginger, turmeric, coriander. Have a light and early dinner. Have your last main meal at least three hours before bed. Do not engage in late-night snacking. If you feel the need for something, sip on a calming herbal tea like chamomile.

∗ Stress reduction: Have a warm bath or a hot shower; put on some nice comfy pyjamas or woolly socks. Light a candle or sit by a warm fire. Do something that allows your nervous system to unwind and relax.

∗ Sleep aid: Create a calming environment in your bedroom with dim lighting and a comfortable sleep environment. Use an essential oil like lavender before bed (spray mist or diffuse in your room) and maybe declutter your bedside locker.

Day 4

∗ Movement: Try some skipping or boxing today to pump the lymphatic system.

∗ Nutrition: Incorporate probiotic-rich foods like yogurt, kefir and fermented vegetables. Stay hydrated with herbal teas or infused water. Cut out processed sugars today.

∗ Stress reduction: Spend time in nature, go for a hike or engage in cold-water immersion (a sea swim or a cold shower).

∗ Sleep aid: Do a guided meditation to facilitate sleep.

Day 5

∗ Movement: Challenge yourself with a high-intensity interval training (HIIT) workout to sweat out waste products and invigorate the body.

∗ Nutrition: Opt for a plant-based day with a variety of colourful fruits, vegetables, legumes and wholegrains.

* Stress reduction: Have a digital detox evening and engage in a calming activity like colouring, journalling or reading.

* Sleep aid: Take a warm bath with Epsom salts to relax muscles and promote better sleep.

Day 6

* Movement: Plan a long walk, a run, a cycle or a hike in nature to boost circulation and lymphatic flow.

* Nutrition: Try intermittent fasting, leaving a 16-hour gap between your last meal at night and your first meal the next day. (Check with a healthcare provider before doing this if you have any specific health conditions.)

* Stress reduction: Engage in a mindfulness practice like guided meditation or body-scan relaxation.

* Sleep aid: Practise gratitude, journalling, deep breathing or saying a prayer to release any busyness from the mind, enabling you to drop into a deeper sleep.

Day 7

* Movement: Practise relaxation exercises to allow your body to recover.

* Nutrition: Eat mindfully, slow down eating, chew your food, say grace before your meals. Give gratitude to the food and remove yourself from the diet mentality, where food is bad or wrong. Instead reframe your food and see it as nourishment and fuel to give your body energy and love.

* Stress reduction: Spend time with loved ones, engage in a creative activity, or pamper yourself with a self-care treatment like a massage, reflexology or a facial.

* Sleep aid: Wind down early by dimming the lights, avoiding caffeine and heavy meals, and practising deep-breathing techniques before bed.

Remember to listen to your body's cues and adjust the schedule to suit your needs and preferences. Balancing the body is not a quick fix and a week-long programme is not the answer for long-term sustained change. You must commit to a lifelong agreement of taking care of yourself daily. However, we must start somewhere and using a weekly schedule like this is a wonderful way to kickstart the body into cleansing, healing, rebalancing and repairing. So let the above be a wonderful starting point to get you going on your journey towards a healthier and happier lifestyle. *(Always consult with a healthcare professional before starting any new exercise or nutrition programme, especially if you have underlying health conditions.)*

The mind balance

This is a process where you focus on decluttering your mind, reducing stress and fostering positive thoughts. By nurturing your mental wellbeing, you will not only support your overall health but also pave the way for a more vibrant and fulfilling life.

* **Decluttering the mind** is as crucial as decluttering our physical space. Just as we tidy up our homes to create a peaceful environment, we must also clear out mental clutter to foster a healthy and calm mindset.

343

* **Reducing stress** is paramount for our mental and physical health. By managing stress through relaxation techniques, mindfulness practices and stress-reducing activities, we can support our mind and improve our overall health.

* **Fostering positive thoughts** is a powerful tool in maintaining a healthy mind. Positive thinking can help reduce stress, boost our mood and enhance our overall wellbeing.

Here's a step-by-step daily practice to help you cleanse your mind and detoxify your thinking so that you can be clearer, calmer and more at ease from the inside out.

Weekly mind balance programme

Day 1: Mindful breathing

* Start the week by practising deep-breathing exercises for 5–10 minutes in the morning and at night. Focus on your breath and let go of any negative or stressful thoughts.

* Options here might include deep belly breathing (page 274), box breathing (page 55), 4–7–8 breathing (page 275), alternate nostril breathing (page 55), cooling breath (page 41), focusing on the flickering flame of a candle, repeating a mantra or simply focusing on the sensation of your breath entering and leaving your body.

Day 2: Gratitude journalling

* Take some time to write down three things you are grateful for each day. This practice can be done at night before bed and each morning on rising. It can help shift

your mindset towards positivity, reduce stress, and act as a brain dump for clearing the mind.

* Take a few deep breaths before starting your journalling session to centre yourself and focus on the present moment.

Day 3: Mirror work

* Look into the mirror and affirm yourself with love and kindness. Look into your eyes and say things such as *I am worthy, I am enough.* Smile at yourself and acknowledge the courage, strength and resilience that you see staring back at you. Practise mirror work as often as you can today, for example first thing in the morning, in the car and again at night time before you close out your day.

Day 4: Guided meditation

* Start your day with a guided meditation. Set aside 10 minutes when you won't be disturbed, find a comfortable position, maybe even light a candle or some incense to create a little sanctuary for yourself. This will help to calm the mind and set positive intentions for your day. If practised at night, it will help set you up for a more restful night's sleep.

Day 5: Affirmations and self-talk

* Start your day by repeating affirmations that align with your goals and values. Write down your affirmations on sticky notes and place them around your home or workplace. Replace negative self talk with empowering statements and speak to yourself with kindness, encouragement and support, just like you would to a friend.

Day 6: Visualisation exercise

* Close your eyes and visualise a peaceful and serene place. Imagine yourself there and focus on the sensations and emotions that come up. Visualise how the best version of you can show up in your day. Visualise how you walk and talk, what you eat, how you move and breathe. Visualise being strong, calm, grounded, kind, peaceful, etc. See yourself as you would like to be today, like watching yourself in a movie.

* Place your hands on your heart and breathe as you do this exercise to further deepen the connection back home to yourself.

Day 7: Forgiveness and letting flow

* Forgiveness towards yourself and others helps to release negative emotions that may be holding you back in life. Today, take a few moments to reflect on any resentments or grudges you may be holding onto. Write a letter to yourself or to the person you need to forgive expressing your feelings and then choose to let go of those negative emotions. Practise self-compassion and remind yourself that forgiveness is a gift you give yourself. Feel the weight lift off your shoulders as you release the burden of holding onto anger or resentment, allowing greater balance and peace to flow into your mind.

Take a day to rest and reflect on the progress you've made throughout the week. Practise deep-breathing exercises as you take time to relax and unwind, letting go of any lingering stress or negativity. Use this day to set new intentions for the week ahead.

This mind balance programme uses many of the tools from the 11 Pillars of Mental Fitness. You can pick and choose the ones that suit you to get started, until they become part of your daily routine. Remember to be consistent with these practices. Consistency breeds change. Change instils new behaviours and thought patterns. Change your thinking for the better; change your world for the better.

The soul balance

Just as we need to cleanse our bodies and minds of stress and impurities, it is equally important to nourish our souls, releasing them from negativity, stress and emotional baggage. Harmonising the soul involves releasing negative emotions and finding flow in our lives, embracing our truth and living in alignment with our core values. In order to do this, we must be willing to release anything that blocks us from living within our heart's space. **We must let go of regrets, grudges and blame, and embrace forgiveness, gratitude and grace.**

Weekly soul balance programme

Day 1: Press pause, reflect and rest

* Start your day (and end your day, if possible) with a 10-minute meditation or mindfulness practice to press pause on life, quiet your mind and centre yourself.

* Take some time to reflect on any negative emotions or thoughts that you may be holding on to. Write them down in a journal and then release them through a symbolic gesture like burning the paper or tearing it up.

Day 2: Surrender and let go

* Let go of resistance and struggles today. Allow things to unfold naturally as they are meant to.

* Pray, connect to the divine, higher source, God, angels, past loved ones, the universe, nature – whatever resonates. Connect, breathe, sigh and let it all go.

* Use the mantra 'For the better' or 'This too shall pass' to help you surrender today.

Day 3: Digital detox

* Disconnect from technology for a set period of time today, starting with a minimum of one hour. Use this time to engage in a relaxing activity such as reading, taking a walk or meditating. This supercharges the soul and tames the 'active' mind.

Day 4: Self care and joyful moments

* Take some time for yourself today and engage in activities that bring you joy and relaxation. This could be reading a book, taking a bath, practising yoga, basking in nature or indulging in a hobby you love.

Day 5: Creativity and expression

* Engage in a creative activity that brings you joy and allows you to express yourself, whether it's painting, writing, dancing or baking.

* Allow yourself to explore your emotions freely through creative expression, letting go of any inhibitions or self-judgement.

* Connect with your inner child and rediscover the innate joy and creativity that resides within you.

Day 6: Connection and community

* Reach out to friends or family members for support and companionship. Perhaps you could go to a community gathering or sign up to a local choir group or running club. Becoming part of a community is key to generating oxytocin, allowing you to connect to a tribe, which yields feelings of safety, security and attachment.

* Volunteer your time or offer acts of kindness to others, fostering a sense of connection and compassion within your community.

* Engage in meaningful conversations and connections that uplift and inspire you, deepening your sense of inter-connectedness with others.

Day 7: Let the divine grace flow

* Connect to the divine grace of love through prayer, meditation, stillness and silence, and let this powerful energy flow through you, filling your heart with love, peace, and gratitude.

* Carve out some time today to sit in this silent space and connect to your soul by asking yourself these powerful questions: What is my soul longing for right now? What would you have me do? What would you have me say? Where would you have me go?

Reflect on your week of soul balance and realignment and journal about any insights, learnings or revelations that have emerged. Integrate the practices and habits that have resonated with you into your daily routine, creating a sustainable foundation for ongoing soul care. Set intentions for how you will continue to nurture and cleanse your soul in the weeks ahead, committing to your ongoing growth and wellbeing.

These weekly schedules for the body, mind and soul are just guidelines. You can tailor them to suit your own preferences and needs. The key is to listen to your inner self, honour your intuition, prioritise the delicate dance between self-care and being of service to the world, and continue to engage in lifestyle habits that honour your whole self and enable you to LIGHT UP.

IGNITE THE LIGHT WITHIN MEDITATION

I hope this book has given you a greater understanding of the deep connection between body, mind and soul and that you have found lots of practical ways to energise your body, awaken your mind and supercharge your soul. To conclude I want to share my Ignite the Light Within meditation. My wish for you is that you use this book to help yourself to truly shine and light up the world around you and I hope this powerful little meditation will support you on your journey. Please use this practice time and time again when you notice yourself shifting back into default patterns or habits that are unserving or unloving. Use this to tap back in and anchor back home. Let your heart navigate you forward; let your light guide you home.

An audio recording in which I guide you through this meditation can be found at www.soulspace.ie/lightup with the password LIGHTUP.

Get into a comfortable position. Drop your shoulders, close your eyes, turn your gaze inwards. Breathe. Settle. Become still. Let the gushing waves of adrenaline and cortisol slow down so that you can activate the healing cascade of hormones and the chemical messengers of growth and repair (serotonin, dopamine, oxytocin) to become elevated, aiding the transmutation of fear into faith, tension into trust, shame into self-care, anger into acceptance, lethargy into lightness, loneliness into love, and perceived weakness into warriorship.

It's time to let the unlived dreams within you blossom into existence. To let your light come forth and be breathed into existence.

As you breathe, reach towards the light. Too often in life we have been told that we don't have the ability to shift, to shine, to change or to grow. We keep our head down instead of tilting it towards the light. As you breathe, you slowly begin to bring fresh oxygen, light, love and hope to each and every cell in your body. You begin to rearrange and reorganise your internal chemistry and biology. Let the stress, strain and struggle, the swirling chaos within, become still and settled. Listen, feel, breathe.

Is there a faint voice within you that wants to rise up and roar? That wants to be heard, seen, acknowledged? Can you listen tentatively, fearlessly, tenderly and graciously? Can you be courageous enough to go within, to dial down the noise, be patient enough to listen and honourable enough to feel?

Bring your awareness down into your heart, which is the altar, the kingdom and the gateway into the soul. Stop, listen to the beating drum, the drum of life, that life-force energy that is living within you.

The soul speaks to us through sensations of the body and through the emotions and feelings of the heart. We place our hands gently upon our hearts. We breathe in compassionately.

We bow our heads graciously towards this anchor point. We find in us a place of quietness. In this place of quietness, we find our strength. We begin to tune in and we begin to hear a new song, a new rhythm, a new tune, a new voice – the beginning of a new story, a springing into life of our soul's script.

Draw your awareness down from your heart into your belly, your solar plexus region, and breathe. Let the fire, the light, the flame burn through all fears, doubts, barriers and blockages. Begin to give yourself permission to activate and reignite this light within. Begin to fan the flames within and let your internal light flicker; let it grow into a beautiful fire representing your passion, strength, courage and power.

This place, this feeling, this sensation is called 'home'. Come home to your heart, to your deepest truths and to your greatest light. As you breathe, remember this place. You are free here – free to create the next chapter, a new song, a new life. As you keep going inwards and reaching towards the light, you begin to emanate and radiate your greatest glow.

ACKNOWLEDGEMENTS

This book has been a huge passion project, a seed that has been germinating for a long time. Without the incredible love, light and support from my loved ones and the team around me, it's safe to say it wouldn't have been brought into existence.

To my incredible husband Gerry. What can I say. You are my hero, my rock, my twin flame. Thank you for your unwavering love, support, inspiration, and devotion. You've held me at my lowest and you've raised me up at my highest. No words can even begin to express how deeply grateful I am for your encouragement in helping me keep finding the light to write this book, and for giving me hope, strength and courage, especially on the days where I doubted myself, my ability or my capacity. Thank you for being the spark that allows me to shine my light.

To my two beautiful angels, Eli and Bethany, my whole world. You have rebirthed me into a whole new existence where I now see life through a new lens. You have become my greatest teachers, my best friends and have revitalised my perspective on life. You are the wings that give me the strength and courage to keep flying high and finding the light.

You light up my day every day and provide me with the most magical of glimmer moments. You make it all worthwhile. Thank you for bursting my heart open in the most unimaginable way possible. I love you both so much.

To my amazing mam and dad. Thank you for dedicating your life to us, for grounding us in values of authentic love and for opening our minds to the bigger questions in life. Thank you for instilling a strong sense of community and gratitude in my life and for always reminding me of what matters most: family, faith and friends. Mam, thank you for instilling in me the love of life, health and vitality, and Dad, thank you for instilling in me a positive mindset and a 'never give up' attitude.

To my brothers Alan and Mark and my sisters Anita and Elaine – thank you for putting up with me for all these years! I genuinely am truly grateful to have you all in my corner, and thank you for always being so supportive and encouraging in all the different chapters throughout my life. You've all guided me in very profound ways and without your kindness and love I'd be lost.

A huge, special thanks to my editors Teresa Daly and Catherine Gough, my agent Faith O'Grady and all the team at Gill for their continued guidance, expertise and faith in me to bring this book to life.

And lastly, to each and every one of you who has picked up this book, I honour and salute you for wanting to reconnect to your soul's script, to find peace in your heart and stand into your light.

NOTES:

NOTES:

NOTES:

NOTES: